I0438378

WINE'S NUTRITIONAL POWER

VITAMINS – MINERALS – ENZYMES – ACIDS

A J MORRIS, JR., PHD

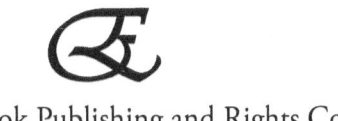

Strategic Book Publishing and Rights Co.

Strategic Book Publishing and Rights Co., LLC
USA | Singapore
www.sbpra.com

For information about special discounts for bulk purchases, please contact Strategic Book Publishing and Rights Co., LLC Special Sales, at bookorder@sbpra.net.

ISBN: 978-1-63135-673-5

Did you know?
Drinking wine feeds more than
twenty-four vitamins,
twelve minerals,
nine enzyme families,
and up to thousand acid complexes
to every cell of a body.

This book is dedicated to the research scientists who have braved the powers of religion, politics, and government to restore the knowledge of the nutritional content of wine—blessed by God from the beginning of time—and to those who stood faithfully behind these wonderful qualities of wine while watching it be crushed asunder by governments and religions. To them I take my hat off!

European nations have claimed wine in their food pyramid. I encourage all, who, today, will restore wine as a food and move it to the top of the US food pyramid. Let me focus special attention and thankfulness to Agnes Fay Morgan, Professor, USDA Research Scientist, Berkley University. In 1938, she published the first official US research on the nutritional properties of wine. She is perhaps the "Founder of American Nutrition" and is an unsung American hero for the wine industry.

Professor Morgan overcame the resistance embedded within the American research community to do wine research. She conducted the first tests that brought USDA-level proof that *wine is a food loaded with vitamins and minerals.* She gave wine its first breath after the "Prohibition Rampage" that burned vineyards across America.

Last but not least, I want to thank my wife, Glenda Sue, for support, vision, and encouragement. Having spent eighteen years in a Biblical research environment, she believed wine deserved serious research and a new consideration. In 1999, we adopted wine for our health.

After much study, the proof was complete, I agree wine is the most perfect food, as Louis Pasteur told us.

Your pastors, doctors, and parents do not know what you are about to learn.

Enjoy!

A J

ACKNOWLEDGMENTS

God Almighty set up wine to be the "king of nutrition"; however, He did not use those words. He told Moses to list "wine" among the foods, including grain, oil, sheep, and cattle, that were His "blessing", (Deuteronomy 7:13). Along with fruits and vegetables, these foods fulfill the nutritional requirements of twentieth century scientific research and form a "food pyramid", the world's first food pyramid.

Moses passed this knowledge and blessing on to us the "modern" descendants but just to make sure we knew the importance of wine, we had another internationally famous teacher called "Jesus Christ, the Messiah," who reconfirmed the value of wine. He did not just teach us, but commanded us, to "remember me" every time we drank the wine, broke bread at the table or did anything and in Matthew 26:27, He said to "drink ye all of it."

We want to acknowledge Hippocrates, the Father of Medicine worldwide, for teaching the power of wine's nutritional benefits as "accelerated healing," which made wine the cornerstone of his medicine. As the gladiator's surgeon, he did hundreds of operations, including two open heart surgeries, which cleansed wounds with wine and sewed them up with certainty that the accelerated "healing" would restore them. This reinforces the most powerful lesson about wine's nutrition in history, by Mnesitheus of Athens, and taught again in two hundred AD by Athenaeus in his book *Deipnosophistae*. Parents ought to listen to Mnesitheus and understand "governments do not obey the Biblical teachings of wine."

"The gods have revealed wine to mortals, to be the greatest blessing for those who use it aright, but for those who use it without measure, the reverse; it gives food to them that take it and strength in mind and body. In medicine it is most beneficial; it can be mixed with liquid and drugs and it brings aid to the wounded. In daily intercourse, to those who mix and drink it moderately, it gives good cheer, but if you overstep the bounds, it brings violence. Mix it half and half, and you get madness, unmixed, bodily collapse."[1]

INTRODUCTION

This research found startling history that explains a great deal about the world conditions of wars, diseases, medicine, and nutrition uncommonly known. All have been manipulated by men, religions, governments, and natural events that could not have been planned by men. You will be amazed to learn how the Catholic Church, the only Christian Church at the time, brought liquor into a place of high esteem after it was discovered in 1225. It became the foundation of Communion in the Church, as the history of Biblical "strong drink" and "liquor" merged to become known just as "wine". The words "strong drink" would lose its place in purifying water of disease. If you can imagine taking Communion with 65–95% alcohol in a brandy, as the manner for remembering Christ, you have a foundation of understanding "confusion within the church".

As a certainty the Little Ice Age of 1341 confirmed the Pope's decision that the Church was supposed to do Communion with liquor because all the European vineyards froze out. As result of the believers being drunk, the Church justified drunkenness as a good thing "because people would trust you." However, it would take 700 years to realize that these drunks were alcohol addicts and not the obedient servants to God, as the Church claimed. No one acknowledged how many addicts came out of this Church theology, which was ordained by the Pope, nor the great spiritual cloak that had covered Christianity. Drunkenness confused kings, produced wars, caused poor leadership, crippled industries, and dehumanized the people.

Theology doctorates could not cure the addicts, nor could they call drunkenness a spiritual curse because it was blessed by the Pope. Secular churches worldwide were under the protection of the Pope. Medical doctors had no authority over addiction and turned it into a money-making machine.

John Wesley was the first Pastor to break the curse, which flooded the world with Methodist Churches full of "teetotalers." Then the Reverend Edward H. Jewett called a debate in 1882 regarding "Good Wine" (no alcohol) vs. "Bad Wine" (alcohol) and determined churches should only serve canned grape juice for Communion. No decision was reached to free wine from the yoke of "*liquor*." The church remained in bondage. The US would go into Prohibition, then decide it was a bad idea, and then go into controlled taxation of alcohol under a federal agency.

This research clarifies the understanding of wine "that it is a liquid food made from the nutritious fermentation of sugars from a juice."

Its acids purify water and kill diseases. Liquor is "a distilled alcohol and has no food or nutritional value." It does not purify water or kill diseases. Next, I encourage the wine industry to identify wine as a food, indeed the "king of nutrition," and label wines with their nutrients printed on the label. Wine is God's foundation for a healthy life.

CONTENTS

CHAPTER 1

WINE POWER

Modern research has found wine nutrients are a complete food. Perhaps this explains why God would include wine in His "food group" of blessings to the Hebrew people, which He named as "oil, wine, grain, sheep, and cattle." According to most of the church leaders I know, not one of them would have seen any purpose for upholding wine as God's blessing in the food plan. They have graduated from the same generation of schools. Do you know people who include wine as a daily family food, like many Italians, French, Israeli, or Greeks do? When the Bible was written, nobody had the scientific measuring tools to know what nutrients were in wine, but as you will soon see, it was indeed their daily multiple vitamin pill.

Do you suppose that when Christ told the apostles at his last supper to "drink of the cup" and to "drink ye all of it" he may have known a multipurpose of nutrition, medicine and spiritual remembrance was important? He foretold the future to his apostles but he did not tell them there was power in the wine—and it is still there! his book of foods we are going to examine the nutritional power e. We are going to discover the vitamins, minerals, enzymes, d foods hidden from our culture. We are the American that was barred from knowing why we should drink at we know what is in wine we can see that Christ had purpose for the wine.

Christ was directing nutritional health into the lives of future believers who were not wine drinkers. He was starting a wine drinking culture among them to produce health and strength and remind the people daily of what his blood covenant is all about.

I believe he knew what he was doing and what modern research has uncovered he did. Wine was given as a blessing to God's people, later to be known as "Hebrews," "Jews," then "Christians" perhaps even before the days of Noah, since we know he planted a new vineyard, down through Abraham and Moses.

> *Deuteronomy 7:13:*
> *And he will love thee, and bless thee and multiply thee: he will also bless the fruit of thy womb and the fruit of thy land, thy corn, and thy wine, and thine oil, the increase of thy kine, and the flocks of thy sheep, in the land which he sware unto thy fathers to give thee.[2]*

In Hebrew "corn" is generic for "grain" and "kine" is generic for "cattle." We learn that these blessings of the Old Testament were carried into the New Testament through Christ—witnessed at the "Last Supper" before his death. This is reported by Paul to the Corinthians to say blessings over the bread eaten and the wine drunk and to remember Christ while doing so. He reported Christ's Last Supper regarding wine as follows:

> *I Corinthians 11:25:*
> *After the same manner also he took the cup when he had supped, saying 'This cup is the new testament in my blood: this do ye, as oft as ye drink it, in remembrance of me.[3]*

The new "Gentile" Christians picked up the blessings of Abraham and Moses. Does this look to you like an accident or more like a big, gigantic plan? Christ's instruction has passed down throug history, but has been warped, twisted, altered, denied, and withheld from the public by governments, kings, clergy, and well-meaning seminaries. We will observe how wine has been a center of money, commerce, taxation, and power—all of which require confusing the public to "stay away from wine." A confused, deceived public cannot benefit from the power of wine. So the benefit comes from learning that wine has *nutritional power*.

God started us out on a vitamin/mineral/acid/enzyme drink called "wine," which had all of these properties of health that no one told us about and now startles us to learn. Our wonderful parents did not know what was in wine. They only knew it had "alcohol" and made people drunk. It would take twentieth century research to show us what is in wine. The research came after wine had been barred from a whole generation of Americans. The research verified wine is for the health of both children and adults. Let us follow a journey of what we have here.

When Christ commanded the drinking of wine "to remember him," he introduced a new thinking among both the Gentiles and Jews. It was not a Gentile custom to ask a blessing at the table when bread was broken and wine was drunk.

The Bible does not tell us what wine does to the body for nutritional purposes. Someone had to research and write this book.

Liquor control through Prohibition was a disastrous mistake by the US Government, but it still lingers upon the American people. Perhaps it is a Biblical curse that remains upon our nation, as many have reported. The wine culture of historical documentation has not been restored to families as the US Congress proclaimed was done in repealing the 18th Amendment. It was not repealed, just reorganized for federal taxation and ATF supervision. The vineyards have returned slowly. The Revenue Act of 1913 provided for taxes of one percent on all incomes above $3,000. Prohibition was passed by Congress in 1918, but not signed by the President until 1920 so as to retain the tax revenue through World War I. During the war,

Congress demanded 77% of income above $3,000 while the US was manufacturing goods for the Allies and Axis. The US Government would not sign the WW I treaty with Germany for three years after the war awaiting repayment. Congress restored the taxes on liquor without losing a step.

It was a new law giving the US Government authority over wine, beer, tobacco, taxes, and liquor, which threw the states into chaos and the confusion of believing they had authority over liquor when all the time it was Alcohol, Tobacco and Firearms (ATF) and the Internal Revenue Service (IRS). It was a money issue and not a drunkenness issue as the public presumed at all. This arm of government would eventually be reorganized into the Alcohol, Tobacco, Tax and Trade Bureau (TTB). ATF controlled the vineyards and grains while the new Food and Drug Administration (FDA) assigned to the United States Department of Agriculture (USDA), controlled the content requirements and fermentation process to the end product.

FDA still refuses to acknowledge the food value in wine and registered it as an "explosive" because it had alcohol in it, which created the Prohibition hostilities against wine. No wine can explode or burn as liquor can when it has more than fifty percent alcohol. FDA mandates beer, wine coolers, and anything under seven percent alcohol, to register food ingredients on the labels. Wine and liquor are claimed to be alcohol and the rich nutrition of wine is deliberately withheld from the American people although it is several times greater than wine coolers, or liquor which has no food content. States control the sales and marketing laws of wine. All these entities are entangled with each other and constantly forcing wineries to clarify regulations.

ATF would use the Catholic definition of wine to include liquor, which has an alcoholic content able to sustain a flame at what is called 100 Proof or fifty percent alcohol. Catholic Communion wine was able to be sixty-five percent until 1896. Wine at thirteen percent alcohol has never been able to sustain a flame and is not an explosive or able to burn. This alone should move wine to USDA food authority.

Wine was orphaned in the warfare. ATF pulled the grapevines out by the roots and burned many American vineyards.

A war for God's blessing and Christ's Communion was before the American people and we had been deceived by pastors, politicians, and big pharma. Knowledge about wine is just now gaining visibility again. Let us observe our Christian origins of wine Communion at the dinner table and pursue the nutrition of wine joyously.

CHAPTER 2

HEROES AND TEACHERS

Searching for the founders, heroes, and teachers in the wine industry gives a surprising foundation. Starting at the top, one has to acknowledge God's contributions of creating the chemistry and telling us he wants us to be in good health. Then Christ, in Matthew 26:27 while telling his disciples to remember him whenever they drank wine makes an unusual command telling them to "drink ye all of it." Great debates have not settled what this meant, but now we have the twenty-first century research showing us the nutrition in the wine. His statement makes sense for the nutrition.

Christ evidently wanted each disciple to drink a whole cup of wine for nutritional purposes because he was starting a new wine-drinking culture for the health of his Church. He is supporting the plan given by his Father. Don't you think they knew that one day we would know that the nutrition was in the cup and understand what they were doing? They would also know that governments, pastors and Popes barred us from nutritional health with laws and regulations to serve big pharma and tax collectors.

We will observe the Greeks had many wine heroes for us, the first being Hippocrates, the "Father of Medicine," who used the accelerated healing powers of wine for treatments of patients, but let's meet our own unsung American heroes.

Agnes Fay Morgan First USDA Nutrition Research Scientist

The story of Agnes Fay Morgan, the first woman to do United States Department of Agriculture (USDA) research at Berkeley University shows us the price she paid for researching wine. She is an unsung American hero to the wine industry. She published her research that wine had food nutrients and it opened political warfare that would prohibit the American people from access to the top food product in the food chain.

I would like to think that wine research is what established Agnes Morgan as the *Founder of American Nutrition*, a peer with Antoine Lavoisier in 1770 for his research in the metabolism of foods. She focused on the analysis of nutrients in foods, the instability of vitamins and proteins during food processing and the physiological effects of vitamin deficiencies. Her research on instability of foods during processing would change American school foods.

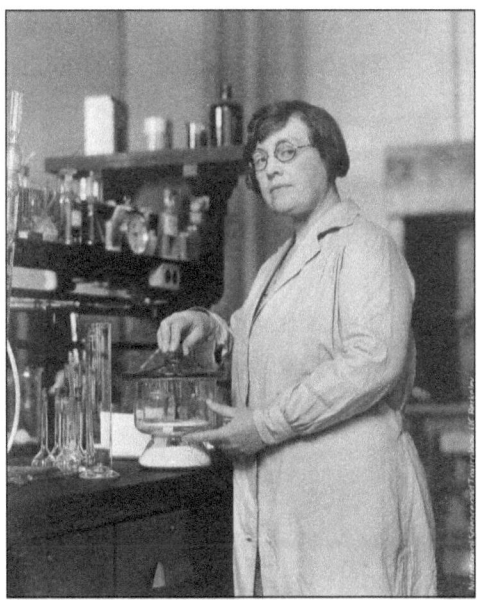

Agnes Fay Morgan, Professor, Director USDA Research, Berkeley University, First Woman to do USDA Research on Wine Nutrition, Established that Vitamins are in Wine.

In 1951 the Iota Sigma Pi Honorary Society for "women under forty" in chemistry created the Agnes Fay Morgan Research Award for Chemistry or Biochemistry. She had "broke the glass ceiling" for women researchers in 1938 as she headed up the first USDA Home Economics, Fruit Products and Viticulture Department of history. Her USDA research should have blown the lid off of the control over wine by ATF and put wine at the top of the American food chain.

Prohibition had thrown out all the public support of wine because ATF defined it as alcohol. They did not distinguish between the fact that alcohol is distilled and wine is not—it's fermented. This is elementary knowledge, but just look at all those that still do not know the difference. Even the American churches did not defend wine and changed Communion wine to juice, a "substitute for wine." But nobody knew anything about wine nutrition until Morgan published the first USDA wine research.

With hindsight we can see from history that she was about to restore the ranking of wine as the leading nutritional food of the US USDA, the largest Bureau of the US Government at that time, was blocked by the power of the American Medical Association (AMA) as wine had proven to also have medical benefits and AMA was dedicated to wipe wine out of the medical industry. Those doors are opening now but ever so slowly. Morgan proved that wine has vitamins and minerals just as the Europeans had reported which fills the research books of Europe. Europeans embraced wine, while the US has never been released from the curse of prohibition. American churches are still locked down.

1938 must have been a year of explosive political war to see who controlled American research and medicine. It was not just a war for truth. FDA was created by the leadership of Royal Copeland, a homeopathic physician and US Senator, incorporated by AIG and put under USDA authority the same year that Morgan published her wine research. Had Morgan's research shown that liquor has no food values the USDA would have provided a great service to America. Wine nutrition should have been an open book showing the path for ATF, soon to become Trade and Tax Bureau (TTB) to control *alcohol* while FDA controlled *fermented nutrition*. This stopped the USDA control of wine as a food. Churches, until this day do not know Biblical strong wine, also called "strong drink," typically ranged from seven to ten percent alcohol, but never over thirteen percent. No Biblical Hebrew ever drank anything stronger than thirteen percent alcohol, which Dr. John Brewer, Wine Master of Wyldwood Cellars in Mulvane, Kansas, reports was the strongest alcohol known to the world before distilled liquor was discovered.[4]

Morgan had the goal of discovering what food nutrition was in all foods and put together a team of researchers at Berkley to identify vitamins and minerals, a great vision for American food and nutrition. She proved the increased nutrition of grape juice as it fermented into wine. She tested both grape juice and wines because the French, Germans and Italians were publishing claims that wines had vitamins not in the juice. She found the grape juice had Vitamins A and C but when it was fermented into wine, it became a wealth of Vitamin B complexes and increased the A and C levels.[5]

Even today it is unknown what "unidentified growth factors" are created in fermentation. Berkley University resultantly did not become the leading institution for USDA nutritional research, and Morgan's research is not in the books where it should be. She has valuable research stored in university records that are hard to find, but those who control the books control the universities. So who controls our books of nutrition? It is AMA and FDA.

Florence Nightingale Nutrition Hero and Teacher

In 1910 Florence Nightingale died and the wine industries of the world heard for the first time that they had a hero, tried and tested beyond all measures, and nobody knew it. Journalist Stephan Luscombe reported "the rest of the story" of what really happened in those barracks in Turkey during the Crimean War where British soldiers were dying by the hundreds every day from one of three plagues. Typhus, Cholera, and Brucellosis were taking down the army. British patriot Florence Nightingale had trained thirty-six nurses along with fifteen nuns and along with her Aunt Kate Smith rose up to help the army.

The British surgeons refused to allow women on the hospital premises. For two months Florence daily requested from the Gener-

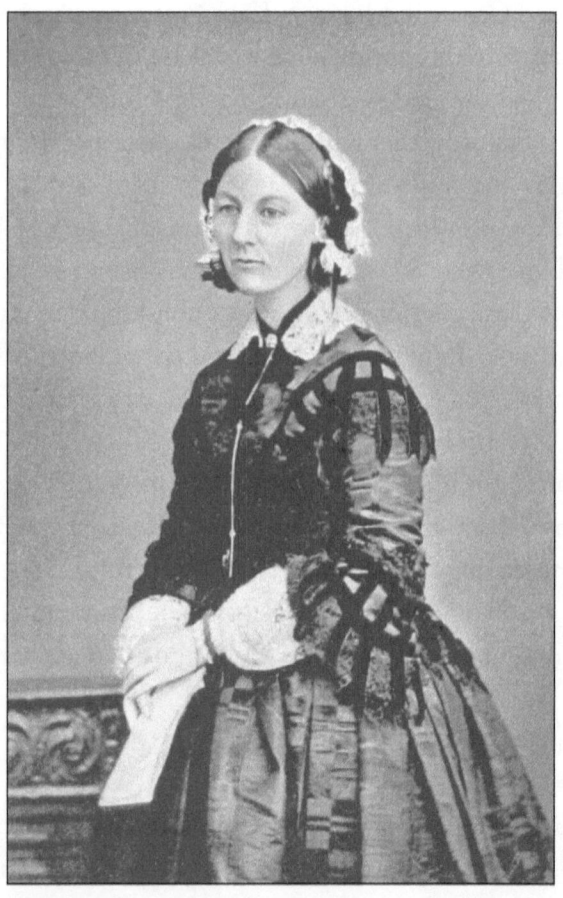

Florence Nightingale, Started Women Nursing Programs, Saved the British Army from Plagues of Cholera, Typhus, and Brucellosis with Wine in the Water Buckets

als the authority to bring her nurses in to help. Orderlies were hauling out the bodies while officers were using the King's best approved medical knowledge to save their lives and losing all of them. We may recall that the Big Book of Distillation became the backbone of British medicine in 1552 and it was a failure. It prescribed treatments with liquor which were Hippocrates treatments with wine. Liquor has no food or medicinal chemistry to heal.

At last, in total frustration at the failure of British medicine, the medical officers rebelled and refused to walk the "floors of the dead". The generals immediately authorized Nightingale to bring in the nurses and nuns but only to haul out bodies and restore orderliness. Nightingale's first action was to put two bottles of wine and a measure of arrowroot in every water bucket. It must have seemed miraculous when the arrowroot stopped the diarrhea overnight and the wine nutrition accelerated healing, which delivered recovery amazingly fast.

The soldiers were cured, literally rescued, and returned to action where the British, Sardinia, Ottoman Empire, and French defeated the Russian expansion across Europe. The British never admitted their medicine did not work, or that Nightingale's remedy did, but they attributed success to Nightingale for bringing order to the barracks that saved the troops. She was acknowledged for establishing women nurses in the medical field and awarded the Merit of Honor by King Edward. Hippocrates would have been proud to honor her for saving the British Army and defeating Russia with weapons of wine and arrowroot.

It would take petri dishes and twentieth century research to discover wine killed cholera in ten seconds and typhus in fifteen seconds. An acidic pH below five killed Brucellosis, cholera, and typhus. All these could withstand high cooking temperatures above 150 degrees and just one time of failing to reach the required high temperature for a meal spread all three plagues. This explains why wine drinkers survive plagues when others die—the nutrition in the wine and its accelerated healing factors rescued the army to win a victory.

So now, we are learning for the first time what is in wine.

It is indisputable that wine is a leading nutritional world food, perhaps the single leading food but American universities do not teach about its nutrition or power. It is still classed in the US, not for its food content, or medical services, but for its alcohol content. What deceptive misleading do the American Churches and people see? This is similar to classing a diamond as a piece of coal instead of the hardest rock or most beautiful jewel known. The glitter and beauty is unperceived. How can we be enlightened in great universities and know so little? Educational control by bureaucrats and big pharma is dangerous.

Wine is not taught for its nutritional or medical properties at leading agriculture universities. Perhaps you think it is a myth that wine was the foundation of world medicine in the books of Hippocrates, the Father of Medicine. This knowledge is still hidden under a cloak of confusion maintained by church doctrines, university book publishers, laws of FDA, policies of TTB, and powers of the AMA medical leaders. How can such a thing happen with the freedom of press in America one might ask? Freedom of press, is controlled in America, anywhere Americans do not stand up and fight for it. It is purely a case of "he who holds the purse strings controls knowledge?" Can you imagine the prosperity and tax revenue America has lost because research is restrained, in every industry? This is not just a wine problem but let's see just how much progress we have made.

CHAPTER 3

WINE'S NUTRITION STOREHOUSE

Wine contains the forty-five nutrients our research industry says are required in a body's nutrition, except for the oil-based Vitamins D and E, which come in cooking or salad oils and would ruin wine. A total of 69 nutrients discovered in wine are listed below by name and hundreds by group. The total may be over a thousand with more discovered yearly.

The storehouse of nutrition was deliberately kept from the American public as result of the prohibition purposes. More importantly, the American medical industry came forth with the new warning "do not drink alcohol" to overcome the traditions that allopath's kept patients drunk and did not heal them. The purpose was to purify their name. Along with this new warning was the twisted definition that wine and liquor were alcohol. It would make no difference that liquor had no nutritional value and was pure alcohol and water. Pedestrians of the street know the difference between wine and liquor. Government definitions of alcohol swallowed up knowledge of a highly intelligent people and barred the American public from wine. It was so simple.

Dictionaries would just redefine alcohol as "any intoxicating liquor containing this spirit," that is alcohol. The 1828 Webster dictionary defined it almost right as "pure or highly rectified spirit obtained from fermented liquors by distillation." This forked tongue definition says wine is a liquor and liquor is a liquor because both contain alcohol, as if distillation was insignificant. So, this is the problem folks. America had organizations of power dependent upon defining wine as alcohol and choking the life out of it. They still have not succeeded. But isn't it strange that both God and Christ would tell us to drink the wine while doctors prohibit it?

Many university reports are flowing into this research as we proceed. It gets more exciting by the year as the precise measurements of nutrients in wine are published. The research money American taxes have paid should have found all this information long ago and disproved that crippling definition of alcohol. Hippocrates told us "one man's food is the next man's medicine." Alcohol is neither a food nor a medicine, but wine is both. How did we get so confused?

Wine may one day show us the foundation of "daily nutrients" required by the body, which are not the international units (IUs) published by USDA. IUs are designed to create sales volumes of vitamins and minerals, not for public health standards. But first let us learn the evidence of what FDA, AMA, WHO, and TTB do not want the world to know. This is the powerhouse that made wine the medicine and food foundation of the world for 6,000 years. This is the arsenal of survival in individual homes that filled the basements, cellars, cisterns, root cellars, family caves, shelter room, and above all wine cellars that have saved millions during and after military raids that burned the crops and storage bins to subdue nations. This is the answer of why wine worked. It stored food. It saved lives. It is the primary proven food of survivalists that saved nations. It is Wine's Nutrition Pyramid. Observe the nutrition:

Wine's Nutritional Source of Power

<u>Vitamins</u>

Vitamin A, Pantothenate aldehydes (B), thiamine (B1), niacin (B3), pyridoxine (B6), cyanocobalamin (B twelve), ascorbic acid (C), riboflavin (G), biotin (H), koagulation (K), Vitamin P, folate, esters, stillenes, resveratrol, hydroxycinnemates, catechins, epicatechins, quercetin, authocyanins, cinnamates, vitisins, pinotins, and portosins are measured. Essential Vitamins D and E are oil-based vitamins and are not found in wine. Oils would destroy the wine.

Minerals

Research currently shows copper, potassium, iron, calcium, manganese, zinc, selenium, sodium, sulfates, sulfites, phosphorus, and magnesium are all in wine. It is reported that regional water tables deliver variations in vitamin and mineral levels that affect the chemistry and taste of the fermented wine.

Enzymes

Pectin Layse, Pectin Methyleserse, Polygolacturonase, Ripadse X-Press, Rapadse Vino Super, Rapadse Ex Color, Beta-Glucanases, Glycosidase, and Cinnamyl esterase are enzymes that are found in wines. Enzyme families are largely unexplained and little is known publically. Enzymes attack and digest foods among their many functions. They also produce the hunger for certain foods which many nations buy before each meal. They know what minerals and vitamins the body needs and tell the brain what to eat. The science of nutrition includes "how to deceive the enzymes" and get them to eat foods not demanded by normal functions. This is used for masking tastes such as using licorice in the feedlot industry to mask molded grains or changes in grains when the prices change for carbohydrates, an agriculture science called "least cost feed formulation". This provides the technology behind taste to entice people to consume "junk foods," hence, the name "consumers."

Acid Complexes

Wine has many acids, producing a pH between three and four. A Riesling wine would have about a 2.9 pH, while a Chardonnay would have about 3.4, with the more sour wine having more acid or the lowest pH. Wine acids will kill many known bacteria, fungus, and virus that the hydrochloric acid of the stomach will not kill which allows a disease into the system. Strangely, the wine acids cause the body to release chemicals that have a higher alkaline pH as part of biological chemistry.

From the Wikipedia Encyclopedia, we find the more common acids in wine are tartaric, keto, phenolic, caftaric, gallic, ellogic, anthocyane, tannic, malic, lactic, citric, succinic, acetic, butyric, ascorbic, sorbic, sulfurous, amineted, ethyl, potassium (some twenty amineted) totaling over a thousand acid complexes.[6] In addition to this arsenal of nutrition, wine has many unidentified nutrients that reportedly aid in the destruction of diseases.

The top three commercial acids of industry are sulfuric, phosphoric, and hydrochloric. They will form acids with metals such as iron sulfate, iron phosphate, and iron chloride and each acid will mix with other acids, which makes it hard to separate them for testing. Because wine has so many minerals and acids, they then combine to form hundreds of acids or acid combinations. The French Wine Guide reported over a thousand unidentified acid complexes are in wine.[7] I have not seen a list.

It makes one wonder if our researchers will ever have the desire to know what balance of nutrition to recommend for a person's body. With the ability to test at the one-part in one-billion parts, the wine industry could and should learn enough to establish a new table of requirements for a healthy body, but someone has to take the lead. All this demonstrates scientific ignorance in our medical industry, ignorance by design.

Carbohydrates and Proteins
From the FDA 1995 Dietary Guidelines for Americans, Fourth Edition, we receive research findings regarding wine's food properties. This research acknowledges vitamins and minerals are in wine,

while announcing it is insignificant in relation to the USDA nutrient recommendations of international units.

The chart of nutrient variations, which is to follow, demonstrates wine has food content even though FDA, at the present time, refuses to allow the wine industry to make food/nutrition claims on the labels. It becomes humorous when you realize that the FDA requires food labels on all beer and wine coolers, because they have less than 7% alcohol, but not on wine labels.

It would seem there is a need to know how much variation is in wines in order to choose a value of one over the other for medicine, nutrition, or just personal taste.

Now let us look at the first research authorized by FDA in 1976 for the world to know about wine nutrition. It is called "Document SR-21— Nutritional Information on Alcoholic Beverage, Wine Table Red."[8] Agnes Morgan is not mentioned but some of this is her research. It did not just report "red wine," as neutral research would have reported. It included the barbs that wine is purely an alcoholic beverage, which may have skewed the objectivity of the research. However, since we have just reviewed the research on the nutrients in wine, these results are confirmation for the American people to know we have been denied real food values for our health by what I'll call "USDA negligence." FDA works under USDA authority.

SR-21 Wine Table Red:
FDA Nutritional Comparison of Alcoholic Beverages

FDA labeled this research as an alcohol chart but liquor is not shown. That is because liquor is distilled and has no food value as wines and beer do. Alcohol has seven calories per ounce of alcohol. However, the chart confirms FDA knows wine has food value and by official means denies wine food properties to the public. It also shows reason that FDA knows wine has medical properties and does not authorize this to be published to the doctors or American people.

Food	Red 12.5%	White 12.5%	Sweet 18%	Beer 5%
Single-Service Size	6 oz.	6 oz.	6 oz.	6 oz.
Sodium	8.5 mg	8.5 mg	15.3 mg	7.2 mg
Calories	123	115	260	319.2
Carbohydrates	2.9 g	1.25 g	20 g	10.56 g
Protein	0.28 g	0.15 g	0.34 g	1.56 g
Vitamin B1 Thiamin	0.01%	0.01%	0.04%	0.0%
Vitamin B2 Riboflavin	0.05%	0.01%	0.04%	0.0%
Vitamin B3 Niacin	0.13%	0.12%	0.36%	1.2 mg
Choline	1.4%	1.2%	1.56%	18 mg
Magnesium	4.0%	4.0%	3.56%[1]	10.8 mg[2]

SR-21 WINE TABLE RED

Nutritional Information on Alcoholic Beverage

Other nations distribute this information to the people for its food value and a different protection system of family health results.

Just the observation of the differences found in this chart gives reasons to choose one beverage over the other, both when selecting one as a food and when putting a price tag on value. As the calorie-counting craze is a deceiving power in the hands of marketing motivators, let us observe that sweet wine has twice as many calories as dry wine and beer has three times as many. Sweet wine has seven times as much carbohydrate as the dry wine, while beer has four times as much. This illustrates why beer drinkers have different body mass than wine drinkers. The nutrients really do change the body. Also one would choose a different beverage based upon the work load demanded of the body. There is real health science in such a small chart of action.

When weight is an issue, we must remember that the body does not have to digest these "foods." They are 100% utilized, which is why both wine and beer have been used as complete foods. They do not give the amount of energy needed for serious work, but both wine and beer have records of being the only food source consumed over long periods of time and the people surviving very nicely in health. In areas where insects and molds destroy the grains quickly, it makes sense to turn the grains into beer. Also beer is easier to transport than grain.

Beer does not purify water nor historically last more than five days before spoiling. Grapes naturally turned into long lasting wine to protect our health and provide food. Wine is a food product while beer is for water replacement and support of work calories.

Dr. John Brewer explained "there are two types of calories in wine, i.e., nutritional and energy burning. There are seven energy-burning calories per ounce of alcohol. For example one pound of wine at ten percent alcohol would have 1.6 ounces of alcohol or 11.2 calories. However, sugar-derived calories are for nutritional body building. Dry wine has no nutritional calories because they have been all turned into alcohol, which is why they call it "dry." Only the sweet wines have energy-burning calories.[9] Sweet wines have nutritional calories. These are the wines to give to a starving or dying man for quick revival from its nutrients. If wines are ever labeled as foods, these decision making values will be on the labels.

Hidden Food Power

In 1997, Dr. John M. Pezzuto, a professor at University of Illinois Chicago, discovered resveratrol was in natural food plants.[10] He had performed many studies on the resveratrol in wine and other foods along with Purdue professors and found startling nutrition and healing results. He set up a collaborative research study with the Purdue University of Biomedical Chemistry and Molecular Pharmacology to evaluate its significance. Dr. M. Jang and a team in joint research with Pezzuto found that cancer received a chemopreventive activity from the resveratrol derived from grapes.[11] Suddenly, in over a thousand government sponsored research studies, it was quickly discovered resveratrol destroyed a wide range of viruses and successfully treated many major diseases with wine as the food source.

This turned the FDA, AMA and HHS laws about wine and medicine upside down. They had built their foundations against wine for its alcohol content which had no medicinal or food values and blocked any research to the contrary. FDA claimed the wine did not produce enough resveratrol to be beneficial but in the course of doing the research a history changing discovery was made. S.V. Penumathsa, Samuel SM, Thirunavukkarasu M, Koneru S, Zhan L, Maulik G, Sudhakaran PR, Maulik N., while conducting research from the Molecular Cardiology and Angiogenesis Laboratory from the Department of Surgery at the University of Connecticut Health Center at Farmington Connecticut,[12] confirmed *wine has resveratrol at significant levels.* This was astounding. They published the results in the US National Library of Medicine National Institutes of Health. It was titled A Promising Agent in Promoting Cardio Protection Against Coronary Heart Disease.

The 2010 Resveratrol Conference held in Denmark reported that some 2,700 published studies were analyzed. They reported 12 mechanisms of action by resveratrol killed diseases of aging, the five leading causes of death which included heart disease, cancer and diabetes while delaying the aging process itself.[13]

This was an astounding powerful result from a historical food and medicine. This answered the age old effective use of wine for foods and medicine by Hippocrates and the DOs. This answered why Christ would instruct Christians to remember him every time they drank the "fruit of the vine." This was the proof that separated wine from liquor. This jerked the rug out from under the medical books, FDA and AMA had created. Wine had a need, a purpose, to be the universal medical and food product in every home and at the Communion table.

As the exciting research comes in, we find one report from Wine Business Monthly that red wine has up to eight times the phenol compounds as white wine.[14] The report is that the muscadine and elderberry wines have the highest resveratrol levels. It is not specific of grape types used or whether the white wine used is just the juice source or the full green grape source. The report defines the phenolic compounds as non-flavonoids, which includes four acid antioxidants. One is stilbenes of the phenol family, which includes Resveratrol. Lastly are flavonoids, which include the flavanols and the anthocyanins. Wine research shows that elderberry and muscadine are the leading grapes for resveratrol content in the wine. Muscadine is dehydrated to make powdered resveratrol and often called "powdered wine," which has no religious resistance for its benefits.

Wine is a food fermented from juices. Liquor is a distilled alcohol and water mixture with no food values. Alcohol is a pure chemical of nature found in foods, especially raw vegetables, fruits and roots.

CHAPTER 4

USDA TRACE NUTRIENTS

USDA International Units of nutrition are not a measurement of the trace nutrients needed by the body each day for health. They simply set standards intended to assure that all the vitamin and mineral companies manufacture and sell their supplements according to a universal scale. What if one Vitamin D company said you needed 1,000 IUs per day and the next company claimed it was only 500 IU, which one would you buy? It was the intent of USDA to provide a standard. But what is an International Unit (IU)? Is it a weight of pound or milligram; a volume of teaspoons or milliliters; a food burning standard of calories, or size such as a millimeter or square inch? It is none of these. The truth is that an IU is not a standard measurement. No pedestrian can measure an IU.

Webster says "an IU is a quantity of a biologic (such as a vitamin, mineral or acid) that produces a particular biological effect agreed upon as an international standard. The "agreement" issue removes all notions this is a standard measurement. Nobody has to "agree on the measurement" of a standard that a millimeter, a liter or a pound are different for each substance measured. Do we tell our children Vitamins A, D, E and minerals are not the same biologic and each one is measured by a different group agreeing? Most Blacks and Chinese cannot digest milk so do we put them on the "committee to agree" on the IUs found in milk? Most Indians cannot digest alcohol so do we put them on the "committee to agree" on IUs of food in wine? Surely we are better than this. We need a viable measuring device.

The "agreed upon" part changes with each substance. So I know that makes everyone feel good because even the experts cannot give you a simple definition. So, I ask you, Mom, how much Vitamin C should you give your ten-pound child, or fifty-pound child, or your two hundred-pound husband? Do you feel competent with IUs? Are we just ignorant or is someone in government standards messing with our brains? Indeed, I have two vitamin companies where one claims twice as much Vitamin A, D, and E are required than the other company does in daily IUs. Both claim their research is the bona fide research for the standards. Interestingly, neither of these agrees with any other companies' standards of how much an IU should be in any biologic. The government standard is not working. We pay taxes to fix this. This is a USDA problem that has gone on for years. Some bright congressman can fix this all by himself.

Animal feed companies mix feeds by "ounce and pound measurements" and they know exactly how much calcium my dog is going to get each day if he eats one pound of food and they do not measure it in IUs. So I am reporting to the human nutrition family that IUs are not a measurement people can understand because governments do not have a clue how many IUs a company sold last year on which to pay taxes, grow animals or give my children.

IUs must be replaced by a measurement people understand. A good place to start is to measure the nutrient levels of wine, which have no conversion loss when assimilated by the body. It is my suspicion that God knew something when He told us wine was a blessing. God's blessing is a dependable measure.

Indeed, companies are not competing on a level table and even the USDA does not know how much nutrient a person really needs. The industry is full of misinformation. Just imagine, we have had thousands of PhDs and professionals telling us for years what none of them can agree upon. Can you imagine a dietitian telling you that every ounce of beet has the same IU of iron no matter where it is grown? They do and they are wrong to tell us that. Some carrots are sweet and others are bitter so everyone knows the dieticians are not given accurate scales to measure. The dietitian will tell you they are the same "because the book says so". However, we want maximum nutrition out of our foods. Doesn't that mean food with measurable life in it? Take a mass-marketed sweet potato and an "organic" sweet potato, put them in water, and see which one will sprout leaves. Why does one appear to produce life and the other is silent—dead—void of life? Don't you think this nutritionally important?

Government agencies work for big industry, not the public. They market by pleasing our eye, our taste buds, and our smelling test to purchase foods. This is big industry profits thinking when it should be family health. So how do we get another Agnes Morgan to do research for us the consumer? That is the job of the USDA and they have a failing grade for all the research money we have given them to improve our health. We do not have a standard system for their performance. With or without vision, corruption or honesty gets the same salary. We do deserve better scientists.

Some 97% of most powdered vitamins and minerals are not absorbed by a body. They are flushed out and excreted by the body, which proves the standard does not give us what the body needs. The USDA is the first to tell us this but they do not solve the problem. My goal is not to demean the USDA standard, but we should fault the leadership for misleading the public to serve industry profits and for failing to know what a body really does need. They have spent billions of our dollars and still do not have this important foundational data. They have the distinction of not knowing the difference between liquor and wine, so they call both "alcohol." At the same time they advise us on weight control, which they alone have built into our nation, with school foods, welfare foods, restaurant foods, and grocery foods and they want us to know we are seventy percent of us overweight. I have known many USDA leaders and agriculture specialists. I like them. I worked with them on many projects. They would be the first to blame government for blocking good health. They know the truth, but they did not write the policies. A congressman has authority to fix this.

Wine nutrients come at trace levels that do not require digesting because they go directly from the wine into the blood stream. They have no waste. They provide greater nutrition to cells than copious quantities of vitamin pills that have to be digested and then pass through the intestines almost unused. Perhaps the worst misconception is that dry vitamin and mineral pills can supply the body with the original acids found in wine. They cannot.

Numerous research centers claim we are wasting our money on dry resveratrol capsules. I have seen no research to the contrary. Liquids are fully digested. Elderberry and muscadine wines have larger quantities of key medical and nutritional benefits than found in most wines.

Just imagine, wine has hundreds of acids usable as food; but vitamin companies cannot deliver a single acid through dry pills. Dehydrated acids do not reconstitute in the stomach just by adding water or body fluids. It takes electrolysis and time to restore dehydrated acids. We have observed this through recharging a battery in a car with electricity. Recharging takes time. The stomach was not intended to digest nutrition taken as dry acid powders claiming to be the genuine nutrients. Without electrolysis the powders just pass out of the body unused.

America has been sold the idea we must take vitamins and minerals because our foods are deficient of nutrition. It makes us paranoid about all our health and food sources to believe this. This was solved by the USDA National Organic Program. It is a worldwide program but in America only has teeth in meats, poultry and egg production which must be 95% natural to be called "organic". This means five percent of all meat, poultry or eggs can be artificial or unnatural products and be called "organic". So much for that standard! "Organic" and "natural" means the product must not have artificial color (we have seen meats with color added), added flavors (salt, nitrates, phosphates are not flavors) hormones (these must be discontinued 72 hours before slaughter), antibiotics (these must be discontinued 72 hours before slaughter) or synthetic substances (sand, dirt, wood, grains, salts, etc. are not synthetic).

The organic labels are for marketing purposes to assure the product is properly labeled for what it contains. "Grass fed beef" may have antibiotics, hormones, and pesticides. Range free and cage free may have antibiotics, vaccines, and pesticides. All natural means standards are relaxed, no artificial ingredients (gmo grains and salts are not artificial) and minimal processing has occurred. "Humane treatment" has no FDA definition. Raised without hormones and no added hormones are not the same.[15] You may look up this program on your web. These are marketing tools that really do get a 20% or more increase in price. Some get 200% to 500% markups from people who believe this takes the risk out of foods.

Many people over 80-years old have never taken vitamin pills and I know some that have never gone to a doctor. They eat out of the same grocery stores we do and never eat the so called "health foods." Why are they healthy if our foods are so deficient? I think most people agree we are deceived about nutrition and have no clue what the real difference is in Health Food vs Walmart Groceries. Perception is our measuring stick and the USDA created the difference to help big industry make more money, not us. Wine is the most reliable food I buy. I know the research of what is in it and it does not change very much because *the food was created in the fermentation process.*

Wine nutrients contain a full scope of vitamins and minerals created by fermentation, all of which is digested.

Other rich fermented foods include sauerkraut, pickles, kimchi, sausages, cheese, sourdough bread, chocolate, coffee beans, and yogurt. They are vitamin, enzyme, and acid rich. Our biology and physiology knowledge is terribly limited and the research in this broad field has been held down by politics, medical journals, and research funding. Hundreds of vitamin companies are trying to duplicate the nutrition that wine delivers. So the vitamin and chemical wars and political powers must prevent the wine industry from getting recognition for the nutrients it brings to the table or they will lose huge profits. Big pharma champions the story wine nutrient levels are unknown. This was historically true but they are now known, and published by modern research. We need to get research at the parts per billion for each ingredient in the wine. However, the complex composition of the acids and nutrients has made it very difficult to get the analysis. Parts per billion, perhaps measured by electron microscopes at a cellular level, is a doable science that breaks through the ignorance.

Historic research from the experience of Hippocrates or Roman and Greek emperors has been conclusive, but they only measured quantities and performance of the wine drinkers. They could not measure ingredients in the wine and had no breathalyzer. But what about the hundreds of tombs of kings that have been opened across Asia and thousands of pottery samples studied by Patrick McGovern.[16] Since wine was the major ingredients he studied in his research on Ancient Wine, we have to presume the kings knew the great medicinal and food values of wine or they would not have been trying to take it into the "after life." Do we believe those experienced by the proof of the ages or do we listen to those still trying to push Prohibition into the hearts of America? We will look into their hearts, as there is a record. But now we applaud the scientific industry excitement as they reassure us with what they are finding.

We know now that bodies do not assimilate all the pills at the same rate for other reasons, such as differences in genetics, health, weight, and GI track. Just as each human body is unique and unlike any other body so are the differences in physiologies. There is no research of how much the body uses, could use, or will use of a food. We all know people who can eat like a horse and never gain a pound, while others convert every morsel to weight gain. Perhaps the food is deficient, but nobody seems to fund a research lab to show what nutrient levels foods deliver.

Agnes Morgan's research served the families of America not the suppliers. Her goals of discovering which foods in the grocery delivered food values did establish the dietician industry. However, the industry was not set up to provide public knowledge about how much nutrition came from the different fields planted. The public has no idea why the carrots of one field are sweet and those from another are bitter, or exactly why one has more nutrition than the next. All apples do not contain the same nutrition, but where are the professional dieticians who should tell us how much they differ by type? Does a green Macintosh have better nutrition than a red Delicious? The public, as a result of dietician and nutritionist failures, has concocted the ideas that all our foods are deficient in nutrition. It is certain this is not totally true and costing our public billions for health security but who knows which crumbs are damaging us?

Most of the world does not take vitamin pills. We should learn from this. They eat foods for health and hundreds of millions drink wine and rich native juices for nutrition. Every decade a new, exotic "fruit juice in a bottle" pops up in the direct-sales nutrition industry that the natives have been knowledgeable about for centuries. America packages it, pasteurizes it, destroys it, and we buy it in the belief it still has the original nutrition.

I believe that measuring the nutrients in wine would give the best standard of nutrients required for health. Since this was God's blessing, where are the dietitians and nutritionists that should tell us what He provided?

America is an herbal nutrition powerhouse, as we can see from the health food stores in every city; but the dieticians and nutritionists are not communicating their research to the public. They do not work for us, the public, who need their knowledge. We have reports from many nutritionists that conflict about similar research. This definitely confuses the public, but generally one is giving a government research study. As government studies have been repeatedly found to promote agendas, I tend to believe the non-governmental reports. However, we have many conflicting governmental reports, and it is fairly easy to determine why they changed their minds.

Digging a little deeper, other reports are usually available to reach final conclusions. Dr. T. Colin Campbell gave us the best answer I have ever heard regarding the possible corruption of FDA, USDA, AMA, nutritionists, doctors, scientists, and government employees that continually give the public bad information on nutrition sciences. He has been the President of the National Institute of Cancer Research for years and his conclusion is "Very few illegal acts need to occur. It doesn't involve large payoffs in secret, smoky hotel lobbies, etc. It's just day-to-day government, science, and industry in the United States."[17] He is reporting the system is corrupt. He is also telling us it is up to us to find truth, and do not listen to government organizations. He is confirming we have no standard by which to measure them.

I have held USDA on a pedestal so long, I just hate it that we haven't had a champion executive show up to lead our great farming potential. I blame the lack of leadership to the fact we only have less than one percent of Americans in farming today. USDA and major agriculture universities have watched as the struggling farmers, using their technology, went bankrupt and sold the farms. This is a leadership problem. When I was a youth, some 80% of Americans were farmers. I think this makes America vulnerable to oppression. If anything threatens our food chains, the natives will go to the farms to find food, but it is imported, and they will not find it.

We were not taught that it was wine that purified the water from streams, lakes, and rivers in Biblical times and made it palatable. The same acids in the wine that purified their water also killed their diseases in the stomach from bad foods. We just do not have a wine culture to teach us this today. As we observe the arid lands of early civilization, we get some understanding that the rivers and streams went dry yearly. Few lakes existed, but springs were truly hallowed and had sweet waters—cities were built around wells.

Modern research now reveals it was the acids in the wine that killed the diseases in the water and health came from the nutrition in the wine. Wine was especially beneficial to the physical development of babies and young people. In America, our youth suffer from many diseases and poor health because they are unprotected. Government has encroached on disabling the families to give proper nutrition and placed health authorities over families to enforce their regulations. As we are in a generation of artificial, petroleum-based, food-and-beverage flavors to entice food consumption through enzyme stimulation, our youth are controlled to consume anything thrown into the preprocessed food vats.

Called "junk foods," the flavors are enticing to both humans and animals, which therein have made them a threat to all health because anything thrown into the vats are legally sold as foods and they are more desirable than health foods. This industry may well have stopped the historical education system for cooking healthy foods. This message was the education I received from Boy Scouts and, as a scout master, taught young boys how to prepare "fine dining on the trail." They carried numerous junk foods and no amount of fine dining was going to overcome junk food, although they did really learn to cook. Junk food was just added to the diet.

Chlorine in the water systems does not protect the children as we perceive. Chlorine is not in the water line just to kill diseases that harm us. It is also there to protect the water line, the pipes themselves, from chemical destruction (calcium, etc.). Chlorine is used to protect us from lead poisoning. Old homes and old city main pipelines used a toxic lead-tin alloy to solder the copper and iron pipes used. Lead has definitely dissolved enough in the water to kill infants and cause brain damage to adults.

Lead is unsafe to animals and humans alike and is one reason for flushing the lines regularly. To overcome lead poisoning in the water lines, chlorine is used to chemically cause a scale to form in the lines by raising and lowering the pH of the water, which seals off the lead joints with a calcium scale. Annually and sometimes more often the scale must be reversed and started over again because the scale will refill the lines and block off all the water. When this is done, the water tastes terrible, and the complaining public will be told something like "the water is turning over in the lake." The taste will come back within about two weeks but all the water spigots that have screens in them will have scale in the screens. We have to remove the scale particles to make the aeration screens work properly.

EPA research reports chlorine in the water causes cancer, which other scientists have reported for years. Our infrastructure needs rethinking. Instead of rethinking, EPA has gone back to its condemning research and claimed the research reports were wrong and that "nobody knows if chlorine causes cancer." This little twist is enough to continue chlorination. EPA has also supported adding fluoride to the water, which causes cancer even faster according to the research. However, the modern alarm is the bromide in the water system, which is claimed to come from the soils naturally, which means they are not responsible for it. However, that is what a water plant is supposed to do…"be responsible for it."

As we watch EPA promote bromine, let me remind all of you high school chemists that the activity chart is Fl, Cl, Br, and then I. Some nations have put Iodine in the water for years and militaries use iodine drops in canteens to kill bacteria. Nobody has tested this iodine for proper absolute water safety, but EPA is playing chemical games for big pharma and we need to know their rules. Ozone water purification is the economic and health answer driving American agriculture to produce healthier animals. It produces healthier humans where it is used.

Many public water systems use ozone purification such as Los Angeles, Paris, Moscow, Philadelphia, and Russellville, Arkansas. Chlorine should be removed from all drinking water before using it. This can be done by letting it set out an hour in an open bowl. Heating it will do the same thing. The chlorine gas will evaporate into the air. Chlorine can be removed by using a simple charcoal water filter like those sold at Walmart or Ace, which should be replaced every few months; and if it is not replaced by plan, it will be replaced when the filter begins to give strange odors to the water. These are not dangerous but that is the clue the filter is contaminated.

Historically, it was not common for people to have diseases regularly as Americans do today. This comes mainly from foods with soil bacteria, fungus, viruses, yeasts, pathogens, etc., which is historical. However, American foods are eaten raw and often not cleaned thoroughly enough, and the soils are the main contamination source. Disease is very uncommon among wine-drinking nations. Wine kills the disease in the water and in the foods in the stomach. Because many people do not know wine defends them, many wine drinking families may skip the wine for several days which does allow the disease to infect them, to slip through the cracks, etc. America's youth have been denied the very substance of nutrition used for health in Bible times. Strong drink was never Biblically offered children or adults, except for those who were ready to perish, as in Proverbs 31:6. Everyone drank the Biblical table wine, even babies, which had an approximate two percent alcohol content.

Laws of Wine

Who could imagine there would be such a thing as natural laws about wine? This is like "gravity causes the apple to fall and leave a knot on your head." The Ancient Greeks told us about the power of wine, which supports the Biblical blessings from God and Christ as they taught that wine is one of the greatest blessings to man. In Leviticus, God said it was His blessing to His people. Let that soak in "HIS BLESSING." Athenaeus, 200 AD, Greek rhetorician and grammarian, wrote *Deipnosophistae,* a book which documented the history of over 800 historians. He supported God's Biblical warnings and blessings. He quotes Mnesitheus of Athens as he reported the common knowledge.

"The gods have revealed wine to mortals, to be the greatest blessing for those who use it aright, but for those who use it without measure, the reverse; it gives food to them that take it and strength in mind and body. In medicine it is most beneficial; it can be mixed with liquid and drugs and it brings aid to the wounded. In daily intercourse, to those who mix and drink it moderately, it gives good cheer, but if you overstep the bounds, it brings violence. Mix it half and half, and you get madness, unmixed, bodily collapse."[18]

This brief description of wine creates what I call "Laws of Wine." It defines wine as one of the greatest blessings to men, and I believe it is the greatest among all foods and beverages. This is proven true by American research. Strong drink was so strong it had to be mixed with water to make it drinkable. Americans drink strong drink which is wine unmixed and do receive bodily collapse when they drink too much. They just go to sleep. Perhaps the "madness" spoken of when one drinks five percent wine all day as the fifty percent mixture with water reports, keeps the nitric-oxide trigger active and causes the body to be super oxygenated and joyous all day, a form of hyperactive. We have never seen anyone drink wine like this all day, so the "madness" is unexplained.

Rome used wine as a battle tactic in which German armies that entered the Roman Empire began drinking strong drink at the ten percent level for replacement of beer at the four percent level. The German soldiers believed they were more macho than Roman troops, who watered down their wine. Their army was soon filled with malcontents, who refused to accept orders from superiors, were continuously borderline drunks, and were easily defeated in battles. This experience quickly explains the four-to-one mixture used by Greeks, Hebrews, and wine-drinking nations.

God's blessing was known and recorded by the history of Greeks, who carried forward Hebrew history. The part referring to the ancient knowledge that "it gives food to them that take it and strength in mind and body" explains why this should be part of our family's nutritional diet. Strength in mind and body sounds good for my family.

Wine is the super nutrition pill. Modern research confirms wine gives nutritional strength. There is no English word for "nutritional strength," so I have called it "accelerated healing." Wine is God's accelerated healing agent in the natural world.

The Greeks say it brings violence, madness, or even bodily collapse. Our world is full of OSHA rules, behavior rules and laws, but for the wine to deliver its own punishment to the violator and reward to the user is masterful. It just sounds like a God plan. If it would teach our children discipline where we fail, then all our children should be brought up on wine. It would give backbone to the family discipline system, sort of like a God plan. It would also teach them to mix the wine with water for health.

CHAPTER 5

WINE DEFINITIONS

We have already observed that wine is not known by the same definition worldwide. However, the Greeks and Hebrews are in agreement. So, now let us track the English dictionaries, Biblical definitions, Greek and Roman definitions, Chinese definitions, Catholic Church "Bull" (not what you think…it's another word for "Laws") and the Rev. Jewett's 1882 debate on "Good Wine" vs. "Bad Wine." These definitions will show us where the confusion came into our cultures and churches.

Noah Webster Dictionary 1828

Wine was (1) the fermented juice of grapes, (2) the fermented juice of certain fruits, prepared with sugar, *spirits*, etc. (3) intoxication, i.e., Noah awoke from his wine, (4) drinking, i.e., they that tarry long at the wine, and (5) a symbol of the blood of Christ.[19] The first defect we see in the 1828 Dictionary is that the word "spirits" (first word for distilled alcohol and water) is used and there were no spirits when the Bible was written. This shows us liquor had become known as wine in America by 1828 qualifying it to be used for Communion. It seems the words "intoxication" and "drinking" both stretch the imagination to "define a liquid substance." Intoxication could be the result of drinking wine, but that does not define a chemical or property of wine. Drinking is

35

an action, not a substance. Webster has made great mistakes the average person can see.

Merriam Webster 1994

Wine is (1) the fermented juice of fresh grapes, (2) wine or a *substitute* used in Christian Communion, (3) a fermented *juice of a plant product*, (4) a *drink that invigorates or intoxicates*, and (5) a dark red color.[20]

We can see a great difference in these two dictionary definitions separated by 150 years. In the 1994 definition, wine could be "made from a fermented juice of any plant product." Fruit juices yes, but leaves, grasses, cane, beets, or potatoes? No. Fruit juices will provide their own yeast to make wine while all the other plants require added water, yeast or sugars to even ferment into beer. We pedestrians know "a drink (all drinks) that invigorate or intoxicate" is not a definition for wine. After all energy drinks, beer and liquor invigorate or intoxicate. By this definition, liquor, beer, and energy drinks qualify for Communion. Common pedestrians know these definitions do not distinguish wine, beer and liquor.

Regarding Communion, how can there be a "substitute" for wine or for any word in a proper dictionary? How can pastors call it "wine" and then acknowledge, as Webster does, that it is a "substitute?" Substituting liquor or boiled grape juice for Communion does not make it wine or fruit of the vine. Dictionaries are weapons that reorganize the whims of governments as reported in George Orwell's "1984." When Webster is wrong, it is for "political correctness" speaking, and we must have truth to save our souls and children. Dictionaries do not make a lie turn into truth.

Biblical Definitions

Let us turn to the Bible again to gain the credible definition we seek. Here we find the word "wine" is used 234 times in the Bible. It gives us ten definitions for Hebrew types of wine and two definitions for Greek. Surely we will find our most needed definition here. There are many more words for descriptive phrases, but we want to know the key nouns. I have provided the Greek and Hebrew words, as well as Strong's numbers and definitions, which aids in authority. Let us number the Hebrew first:

1. *Enab* H6025 is the fresh moist grapes when they are first picked and eaten or put into the wine vat. They have the juice that makes wine and it begins to ferment the minute it is picked from the vine and sometimes even before picking. We have all eaten fully ripened grapes that had the fermented taste and were very sweet.

2. *Tsammuwq (yabesh)* H6778 is the dried grape or raisin, which has sugared and is fermented slightly. All raisins have slight fermentation. Raisins can be added to wine and re-fermented to make sweet wine and increase the alcohol content up to 13% for longer life. Alcohol is wine's preservative. Wine must have over ten percent alcohol to endure over time and not turn to vinegar. Exported wine must be over ten percent. The yeast and sugar interaction of many grapes will not produce ten percent alcohol according to Wine Master Dr. John Brewer.[21]

3. *Tiyrosh* H8492 has a range of wine processing, typically two weeks at about 70 degrees or longer at cooler temperatures. As it ferments creating vitamins, enzymes, and acids, it increases in alcohol from zero to up to thirteen percent depending upon the yeast used, the temperature, and the sugar in the grape. This is typically called "new wine" and is very sweet from the flavor of the fresh fruit. It is delightful and easily causes drunkenness because it is constantly getting

stronger—one day you could be drinking a one percent wine and the next week a thirteen percent strong drink when fermentation of all the sugar is finished. When fermentation is finished it is also "strong drink." It will take time even after the sugars are completely fermented out before the fresh grape flavor is gone.

4. *Shekar* H7941 is strong drink when all the sugar is fermented in *tiyrosh* and the sweet flavor changes to dry. It is the typical western dry wine. As wine gets older, the fruit impurities settle out and the wine acquires a refined flavor, which qualifies it as *yayin* or banquet wine. Filtering wine with clay or fine microfiltration is used to accelerate *yayin* quality, which was worthy to be poured as a drink offering unto God in Numbers 28:7.

5. *Cobe mahal* H5435 & H4107 is the name applied when new "*shekar*" (strong drink) is used for the daily drinking and not yet refined to "*yayin*" *banquet* wine.

6. *Yayin* H3196 is banquet wine, old wine or fine wine. This comes from aged "*shekar*" in which the "fines" (the old dead matter) of the grape have separated fully from the strong drink. It is the best of the best.

7. *Chomets* H2558 is vinegar. Wine turns to vinegar when it is exposed to oxygen in the air. The alcohol in the wine chemically turns to acidic acid, which is vinegar. Typically bad wine, which is seven to ten percent alcohol turns to vinegar which has the full range of minerals, acids, enzymes and vitamins of wine but will destroy enamel on the teeth. FDA does not allow publishing the food value of this Biblically acclaimed food.

8. *Mamcak* H4469 is mixed wine with fruit juices, herbs, spices, honey and water for social drinks. It keeps drinks free of disease without ice.

9. *Mishrah* H8281 is steeped hot wine such as a favorite sherry before bedtime or when coming in from the cold. It is primarily used for preventive medicine and nutrition.

10. *Aciyc* H6071 is the "*must*" or hulls, stems, and sticks from which the juice has been squeezed. This "must" may have water added to make a sweet drink before it is passed to become animal feed or fertilizer.

All these definitions are found in the Old Testament, which is written in Hebrew. Now let us observe the New Testament, which has three Greek words defined as follows:

1. *Oinos* G3631 is a broad spectrum word for any kind of wine from the fresh grape to the old wine. This definition includes the water and wine mixture in the mixing bowls that ranged about two percent alcohol for the families.

2. *Gleukos* G1098 is the new wine, sweet and easily inebriating as it becomes strong drink. It is fermenting juice sugars ranging from zero to thirteen percent alcohol.

3. *Sikera* G4608 is strong drink, the same as the Hebrew word "*shekar*."

Greek and Roman Definitions

We have just learned the definitions of wine in the Bible so now we can see why the most important definition of wine is missing from the Bible. The Greeks and Romans gave us the common definition of the ages. The definition of "*wine*" is "*one part strong drink mixed with one or more parts water*." There is no place in the Bible that instructs the mixing of strong drink and water to create "wine."

Greek history speaks of a "mixing bowl," which we would call a "water bucket," where *Cobe mahal* wine was mixed for daily consumption. Perhaps this was such common knowledge that God did not need to define it. The customary Hebrew and Greek mixture was one part strong drink to four parts water. The Romans mixed one to three and the history books of the age's shows great arguments for the right mixture to make wine. Wine would keep its taste when mixed with bitter medical herbs, honey, fruit juices, cinnamon and many flavors not practiced today. It was the center of hospitality.

Hippocrates, The Father of Medicine, in 400 BC, used different wines for treating different diseases in his medical books. Many of his treatments were nutrition based. For example sweet wines were used for the starving, which provided the rapid recovery through sugars, which dry wines would not have delivered. However, all the wines would purify the water and produce palatable tastes. Wine works in the stomach just as easily as purification in the mixing bowls for disease control.

Chinese Definition

The Chinese call all liquors "wine," I mean moonshine quality, 190-proof alcohol is "wine" in China. Rice wine is liquor made from grains that may include rice. When distilled liquor moved across the world to replace strong drink in 1225 AD (discussed in detail in Chapter 7), Asia named everything that was fermented or distilled "wine" following the Catholic Church lead. Chinese wine is not used like Biblical wine for Communion, or as a water purifier, or nutritional food product. Their wine is designed for many toasts at formal dining. The sizes of wine glasses throughout Asia are very small, perhaps gauged to the alcohol content of the wine produced in a region. I never saw a Chinese businessman or official drunk after a banquet although I saw many red faces.

Knowing that the worldwide definitions of wine are not the same helps us understand how governments make different laws about wine. Still, one would think Christianity would have one doctrine about wine, but we can now see that other nations do not agree with American wine laws, which are the same as liquor laws. America is on its own path and needs to refine the definition of alcohol which is "a pure chemical." Wine needs to be redefined as "the fermented drink of fruit juices" with no additions of water, distilled alcohol, acids or sugars.

As I visited China doing joint ventures and research, I found that "boiled water" was and is Asia's water purification system, which causes their industries to have tea three to five times a day. They do not have public drinking water systems. A hot water pot is in every office with tea available for all. They do have public water, but not for drinking out of the tap. They boil water from the municipal delivery system, which is not chemically contaminated.

The health standard set by Confucius in China about 500 BC was *that all water must be boiled before use and all food must be cooked.*

The public ordinances set up by Confucius still control Chinese laws and municipal exams. He was not a religious leader but was appointed by the Emperor to establish organization of governments, counties, cities and municipal health. This also made him a judge. The power of Confucius still binds Asia together through the health laws and government organizations but especially with water purification in the homes.

Did you ever wonder why raw salads entrees are not on the menu in a Chinese or Asian restaurant? Chinese do not serve the American five food groups. I never ate a raw vegetable or salad over the two years I lived in China. Confucian health law says, "Do not eat anything that is not cooked or boiled." Every Asian child is taught this by age two. The result is stir-fry foods that are heated just enough to kill the diseases, roughly 165 degrees on the outside of the vegetables. Interestingly this is roughly the method of freezing vegetables taught by the USDA.

The European and US cultures eat fresh uncooked vegetables by government instruction. They get diseases from raw vegetables due to following government ordinances and doctors do not know to stop it. However, it creates patients. Why would raw vegetables be on the food pyramid if they give us diseases? Disease makes money and creates medical needs for the doctors. People are allergic to many of these raw foods and we have not changed since Socrates reported "One man's food is the next man's poison." I used to be highly allergic to tart citric acids, radishes, cabbages, shell fish, lobster and a few strong cheeses, which caused indigestion and made my mouth break out. I am thankful to be able to eat most everything now. Allergies change with age.

Cooked foods change poisons, just as freezing many fruits make them sweet and the birds know when they can eat the poison berries after freezing. However, milk products of which forty percent of Americans are lactose intolerant cannot be changed. Those who drink wine do not get diseases from raw foods. If they drink wine, the disease does not harm them. If they do not, they can have food poisoning, flu, viruses, and fungus, which cause sicknesses that wine destroys. The very best washing and cleaning standards of USDA and FDA do minimize our disease…but it is not 100% safe as their reports show us. We need wine's protection and there is no substitute for it. Our children deserve knowledge.

American Definition

Liquor was in full force defined a wine and used for Communion in the churches when America was discovered. America had pure water and millions of fresh, pure springs, which Europe and Asia did not have. Perhaps God intended for the new world to learn about wine from its own research. What would be the most valuable crop in the world if everyone used wine to purify their water? The world would be full of vineyards and some nations are! Many countries still have vineyards for water purification and would reject chlorine.

We never had a Biblical "wine culture" in America because liquor was discovered before America was discovered by Spain and had become a Catholic Church staple for Communion. Unlike the beer-drinking nations of Europe, America went after liquor and beer for the alcoholic effects because we did not need either for hydration or wine for purifying the water. Churches had already accepted distilled liquor for Communion. Drunkenness was a Catholic Church blessed condition tolerated by Angleton Churches and other religions as cultural heritage of America. The "liquor culture" flourished as it was cheaper than grape wine for Communion and could be made from any type of grain or juice that were fermented and distilled. Liquor did not have a shelf life for going bad. Liquor caused intoxication quickly and could be mixed with many juices and flavors as the center of hospitality. The definition of wine included liquor and the definition of liquor included wine. The 1828 definition of liquor included milk, blood, sap, juice and any distilled or fermented fluids. However, the 1828 definition of alcohol was a distilled substance from a fermented fluid. So here is a source of confusion. Communion wine was definitely not distilled in Christ's time. The definition of wine had been corrupted to include liquor, but the definition of alcohol did not include wine. It included the liquor made from wine. Governments and religions have entangled wine with liquor. Christ's commandment only applied to drinking wine for Communion. The churches have moved far astray.

The wine industry is very sophisticated with some 1,800 different yeasts and flavors to ferment the juices. These have a range of alcohol content that runs from about seven to thirteen percent alcohol. It takes ten percent alcohol to protect the shelf life of wines for more than a year unless refrigerated. Some wines have a higher alcohol content supplied by mixing distilled liquor to the wine as it finishes fermenting. Dr. John Brewer who is an international wine judge, a wine making master, and owns Wyldwood Cellars Winery, the largest elderberry winery in America, claims the wine industry is so advanced that he can make any "named flavor" of wine in the world just because he knows how to use the yeasts and quality grape technology. This is a great benefit to wine drinkers.

CHAPTER 6

WINE SCIENCES WE NEED TO KNOW

We learn from T. Leary that "Wine is a whole food, the most readily digestible food substance known to science."[22] He provides this in his conclusion of the United States Department of Agriculture (USDA) research that shows vitamins, minerals, enzymes, and acids make up wine. The USDA has the research that wine is the most digestible of all food substances and yet does not shout this wonderful message to the keepers of health or pillars of the food pyramid. Just because it is in some obscure print does not make it a pillar of knowledge. Someone has to teach it. People must demand the acceptance of wine as a food in order to integrate it into hospitals. Why not serve those who are weak the best food known to man, a food that accelerates healing, protects families, and a food that builds Olympians for a nation?

Red wines are fermented with hulls, juices, pods, seeds, sticks, and stems together for the first two weeks and resultantly have a higher mineral and nutritional content than white wines. Modern research shows that the white wines generally have a lower concentration of some nutrients, vitamins, or acids than the red wines. The squeezed juice of red grapes makes white wines but they cannot be fermented with the hulls pods, seeds, etc. There are also green grapes which make white wines when fermented with the hulls, pods, seeds, sticks and stems. However, white wines are typically gentler, sweeter, and more delicate for nutrition than the red ones. This results in white wines being the favorite of women (most of them anyway, my Glenda Sue likes the dry reds).

Research shows the effeminate society is the largest buyer of wine varieties. Wines are drunk worldwide for safety against diseases. Many people claim they do not like any wines and I can assure you that they have not tasted the wide range of sweet wines and flavors available, some 1,800 of them times all the varieties of grapes, and I doubt anyone can tell us how many that is. I did not like the first wine I drank and it was a dry red wine. Dry wines seem to require a developed taste, but after learning the nutrition and health values of it, I stepped forward and now like most every wine for its uniqueness. I still like the sweet wines best and the fruit of the American muscadine is the best of all flavors to me. However, the diabetes association only approves drinking dry wines because all the sugar is fermented out and that is their critical restriction. Diabetics are free to drink dry wines.

The Bible and history books have reports from many nations about the good health and strength of the Hebrews. They believed good health was supernatural from God, but modern research has shown their secret was all the vitamins, acids, and minerals in the addition of wine to the diet. Even today, scurvy, rickets, and malnutrition continue to plague many nations, especially hot and dry lands. The British were called "limeys" because when at sea over a month, their sailors had scurvy from Vitamin C deficiencies while the French and wine-drinking nations did not succumb. The British Navy used limes and three fingers of rum to overcome the scurvy and rickets in the cold weather of the North Atlantic.

The preeminence of wine as a "perfect food" was taught by Frenchman Louis Pasteur, the Father of Germ Theory and the Father of Bacteriology. His statement was, "Wine is the most healthful and hygienic of all beverages."[23] He also claimed, "Wine was the closest known substance to blood."

Pasteur fathered all the vaccines of the USDA yet we did not follow his wine research. He did not define the minerals, vitamins, acids, or nutritional properties, as they were still not known as the building blocks of food, but he was a pioneer leader of USDA laws. The most perfect food is not taught to U.S. families as it is in other nations where food costs are a family economic pillar of life. Wine is recognized as the top of the food chain in most nations. Americans pay more for vitamins or junk foods than the low costs of wine for nutritional purposes. Further, they do not know they can make their own wine. For example, during Prohibition, a favorite way to save the vineyards was to contract with neighbors that they would buy so many acres of grapes and make their own wine. These contracts kept ATF from pulling the vines and burning the vineyards, but many did not learn early enough how to save their fields and their hard work.

Dr. Paul Okunieff, Chief of Radiation Oncology at the James P. Wilmot Cancer Center, at the University of Rochester Medical Center, is the first researcher to tell America that wine should be a hospital food, and he finished that research in 2008.[24] Research was overwhelming from other sources, but it takes a bold doctor to step out and say something so revolutionary. Wine was the major hospital food for two thousand years before it was shut off by government law and religious theology. Now, for the first time, scientists are telling us again that wine belongs in the hospitals. It is the master of nutrition.

Using wine for transfusions may have been the best life source ever used for emergencies. Compare the rich foods and acids in wine to the simple plasma of blood in a transfusion which has no food value or ability to kill diseases. Compare the Vitamin K that stops bleeding to plasma that has no way to stop the bleeding. Both military and family doctors have used wine for transfusions and saved lives, but they feared the Church and medical fathers would imagine something was wrong with putting wine in the blood stream. Neither ever gave an official position about using wine for transfusions, but it was used in emergencies. However, it is so cheap that big pharma cannot make any money from it today and have put a requirement that all transfusions must have a pH of seven, which knocks the acid complexes of wine out of acceptability. Wine is a pure and unadulterated life-saving transfusion, which researchers have been unable to duplicate to this day.

Can you imagine a perfect food that gives rapid recovery to hospital patients, and today's doctors do not know their medical ancestors used it every day? We are not taught that we are supposed to get well "quickly" in the hospitals. This accelerated healing is within the power of doctors. American medical schools do not teach the arts of accelerated healing. Nutritionists and the medical staff of this century are afraid to provide wine as the food of choice to the sick. We have the US Food Pyramid, which does not include wine, but the food groups of other nations include wine.[25] We see in the "Images of Food Pyramids of the World" that France, Germany, and Italy show wine as a foundation of good health. The US Food Pyramid was formed after Prohibition, which may explain wine's absence from the food group. India lists wine in the "Twelve Foods of India."[26]

If a person in the US were asked, "What is the most perfect food?" they would likely respond "milk." Europeans would say, "Wine." Asians would likely say rice. America's information comes from the USDA advertising of milk for years, along with the milk industry promotions. However, modern research shows milk produces constipation in some forty percent of the US population due to lactose intolerance and close to 100% in many nations. This is especially disabling to Black and Asian cultures, which do not have a milk heritage. Medical doctors are taught about this, but it brings patients back many times if nobody tells them to stop drinking milk. Doctors cannot teach against the school milk program. This is such a little thing and US doctors know the problem. This is a poor certification of a whole professional industry, and they can stop it, but it would collectively cost doctors, hospitals and exlax products billions, but milk industry hundreds of billions.

All my children, Jonathan, Melani, and Kristen, were lactose intolerant and could not keep down homogenized pasteurized cow's milk. Can you imagine my anguish in watching my children spit out what I believed was their life force? Millions of you have watched this. We thought it was sickness and spent a ton of money trying to discover what was wrong with them. Raw milk may have avoided the problem, but it was illegal to buy. It had to be pasteurized. Not one doctor (and we took them to three different ones), told us this well-known fact. Instead they put my children on Similac and Mulsoy (neither of which worked), both of which are still being recommended today.

Milk substitutes are industry products to make money, to heck with my children and yours. In desperation, we shifted early to baby foods. Perhaps FDA does not allow doctors to give any other answers. This injured my family and may have affected their life-long health. I hope not. It proved to me the medical education of our American doctors leaves out important information and has them hawking industrial products. I suspect this is why so many doctors have become mavericks and gone back to other medical professions.

American schools give all children the ever-promoted cow's milk when statistics are known that forty percent cannot digest it, hate it, will not drink it, and put it in the trash. Many are sick in the classroom after lunch from drinking milk, as they go through the allergic reaction. Teachers most likely misidentify the allergic reaction because nobody has taught them why the attention span drops so drastically. They grade the students down and nobody stops the system. However, USDA recommends milk in the food pyramid knowing they are damaging forty percent of our children and families. Today, research shows that goat's milk has solved this problem for millions of families and that it digests in the stomach within twenty minutes while it takes ten hours for a child to digest cow's milk. This affects school performance. However, after doing this research, I would now do what millions of parents have done before me and would give my children diluted strong drink, which was the Biblical answer all along.

Nitric-Oxide Trigger that Produces Joy

As we learn more about scientific research into wine, we can observe that within two minutes from drinking the first sips of wine that it begins to relax and lighten the attitude. Soon joy and rejoicing are easy in the conversation. Strains of the day evaporate. This is too soon to react to alcohol. Relaxation is less likely to occur with beer or liquor, which often depresses a person or causes high-stress reactions. This wonderful, gentle relaxation is not from the alcohol in the wine, as Americans would suppose.

> *Zechariah 10:7:*
> *And they of Ephraim shall be like a mighty man and their heart shall rejoice as through wine: yea, their children shall see it, and be glad; their heart shall rejoice in the Lord.*

It is Biblical that one gets joyous from drinking wine. Alcohol from beer and today's liquor are not as fast as wine in producing a physiological effect. Have you ever noticed there is a different time schedule? Neither beer nor liquor produces joy and rejoicing. Few know why. Even your doctors do not know why because nobody taught them in med school. Beer and liquor must wait for the alcohol to deaden brain nerves before an effect becomes observable which may be 20 minutes or more. Wine drinkers know this effect is very rapid, but, like their peers, believe it is the alcohol. Therein, wine drinkers have always believed it was the alcohol in the wine that made them feel good. Only since 1998 could anyone know for certain what the cause for feeling good was. Women tend to be in tune with this physiological effect more than men, which explains why more women than men drink wine. Women know their bodies.

Although many knew the effects of wine were different than those of beer or liquor, none of the psychologists were taught this or how important it could be for emotional therapy. By releasing and enlarging the blood vessels the food particles, dead cells and debris in the vessels are flushed out of the body. Immediately this is replaced by large supplies of oxygen which provides aggressive antioxidants while creating the refreshing harmony of joy. There is nothing like this physiology in carbohydrate based liquor or beer.

In 1998 a Nobel Prize in Physiology or Medicine was given to Robert F. Furchgott, Louis J. Ignarro, and Ferid Murad for discovering "the nitric oxide as a signaling molecule in the cardiovascular system" also called the nitric oxide trigger. This trigger relaxes the muscles that surround the arteries and blood vessels, which causes an instant release and a lowering of pressure on the heart. Wine creates the nitric oxide and releases the trigger just as a nitroglycerine tablet does for heart patients. This explains the Biblical joy from drinking wine. It begins within just a few minutes of taking that first sip of wine.

C. T. Kappagoda, M.D., a Cardiologist, explained in 1998 "…a critical feature of red wine is that it has metric phenolics, which produce a nitric-oxide trigger to the endothelium. This causes the arteries to dilate for a short period of time. When the nitric acid in the wine hits the tongue, the trigger is activated. "[27] Listen to that! "When…the wine hits the tongue…." Wine relaxes us quickly. This causes all the muscles that surround the arteries to relax, which enlarges the vessels. The blood immediately flows through the body without any resistance. This filters out food and dead cells. Even better, it carries a full load of oxygen into the body. The blood is cleansed. Then flushing the body with oxygen energizes a person and makes them feel good. This causes the joyous result the Bible reports.

In the nineteen seventies, Dr. William Beeson, Dean of Nutrition, University of Kentucky, gave annual speeches during the time I worked with American Broadcasting's animal feed industry. I had heard him talk about the "unidentified growth factors" found in the manufacturing of liquors and beer, resulting from the fermentation process. For three years I heard him announce that the best research team in the animal feed nutrition industry could not discover what the "unidentified growth factors" were. He reported to the National Distillers Association members about the *unidentified growth factors* (i.e., low-level vitamins, minerals, acids, and enzymes) in dried distiller's grains that promoted growth of animals much greater than the grains would do by themselves. Dried distiller's grains are the grain products left over after fermenting grain starch out of the corn to make liquor. Even after taking the sugar carbohydrate out of the grain, which is the main benefit of corn, animal feeders will pay a twenty percent higher price for the fermented grain than for the corn alone. They love adding dry distiller's grains to their cattle feed.[28]

Fermentation makes a gigantic change in the food value of corn starches. It is full of new vitamins. Fermentation is a food-production system. It creates vitamins, enzymes, and acids in the corn as a food. For the third time, I heard almost the same speech. Dr. Beeson continued to say, "We do not know what these unidentified growth factors are." Only after doing this wine research did I realize that he was blocked by FDA and ATF regulation from reporting the many acids, enzymes, and vitamins that were created in the fermentation mash of liquor. He could not report that fermentation produced food. However, the feed industry is not fooled by the FDA and ATF regulations. They measure their production in real dollars caused by the increased weight of the animal. Distiller's grains definitely have measurable value for use in animal feeds.

Today, some of the most successful beef feedlots use feed that is predominately distiller's grains and alfalfa hay to make an exceedingly tender steak. In other nations, the grape "must" (left over from fermentation) is added to feed for beef animals. TTB forbids this in US vineyards because TTB controls animal feedstock. Unlike the liquor and beer industries, which sell its mash for animal feeds, wineries have to spread the must back into the fields, which gives international wineries and American liquor distillers an economic advantage over American wine growers' costs. It raises the costs of American wine with no added value. At the same time because beer is less than seven percent alcohol, FDA requires the beer industry to show on the label how much food value a beer or wine cooler gives the drinker, but it's not required for wine.

We have research on the Kobe beef of Japan. The animals are raised on nothing but a beer and mash diet that produces what is touted to be "the most tender and flavorful beef on earth." I am confident many world beefeaters and American feedlots would fuss with this claim in a real test, but the point is that fermentation creates nutrition and the Japanese use it to produce good beef. TTB does not allow wine must to be fed for animal feed, as it is worldwide. This gives an unfair advantage monetarily to international wine producers over the US because they cannot profit from their must.

America has veal grown in similar specialized feeding programs and Jewish pride is taken that their people only eat "the best" beef when they eat "prime" beef. Kobe beef was sold on the world market in June 2014 at somewhere between $400 and $500 (US dollars) per pound. Not only did they refuse to export the Kobe beef until about 2006, Japan refused to import American beef and has succeeded in controlling the politics of this pricing game for 200 years. I have never seen research that compares nutrient values of Kobe beef and doubt there ever will be such research. However, this example of beef politics explains how wine has been maligned for so many years in the US while foreign wine producers have an edge over American wine producers.

P.A. Norrie tells us in his scientific and historical research that "hospitals used wine as a medicine in the middle ages. The single biggest expense at Leicester Hospital of England in 1773 was wine for the patients." He reported that "Alice Hospital of Darrneta, Germany, used 4,633 bottles of white wine, 6,332 bottles of red wine, 630 bottles of port and 60 bottles of champagne for 755 patients in 1870." [29] The nutrient values of wine account for rapid recovery and doctors had no idea what nutrients were in the wine— they just knew it worked. This was common medicine that America did not use.

According to the French Connection Reports, wine has over 1000 acid complexes that provide critical nutritional elements. It is reported that these acids digested foods more thoroughly than hydrochloric acid in the stomach. In addition, they destroyed perhaps every bacterium known to man and unknown diseases.[30] This report also provided comprehensive listings of nutrients in wine, which included every elemental nutrient required for the body except the oil-based Vitamins D and E.

Dr. Mercola's reports (and medical research journals confirm his reports) that what is called the "The French Paradox" explains the value of wine. He cites the 1991 report by Dr. Serge Renaud, a French Doctor, remarking on the health of the French, that they drank wine, ate large quantities of fat foods, and remained thin, that they had better stamina and heart rates than world peers, all explained by the consumption of red wine.

The food miracles of The French Paradox was reported on "60 Minutes" in 1991 to thirty-three million US people, which resulted in a reportedly forty-forty percent increase in the consumption of wine in the US The critical element was that they had better cardio-vascular health than otherwise healthy people who did not drink wine.[31]

CHAPTER 7

THE LIQUOR BOMB

In 1225, spirits were discovered as a result of distilling wine with the new "Alembic Still." The "Alembic Still" had been invented by an Arab named Jabir Ibn Hayyan around 810 AD, an invention that would name him the "Father of Chemistry" to the world. However, an articulate Franciscan Monk, Raymund Lull, established the power of the still when he announced the still's "spirits," made from wine, which would become a "bomb blast" heard around the world. Lull would get Papal support for this new drink he called "aqua vita," the "water of life." He claimed it was "an emanation of the divinity, an element newly revealed to man, but hid from antiquity because the human race was then too young to need this beverage, which is destined to revive the energies of modern decrepitude." He electrified the world with strong, intoxicating distilled spirits.[32]

The Catholic Church acknowledged this new super wine called "spirits" in a Bull (Law) that replaced strong drink in the Communion cup with distilled liquor. Can you imagine that? They began drinking liquor for Communion instead of wine, plus the people stopped pouring wine in the mixing bowl to purify their water and started mixing this distilled "super wine" in the water. Distilled alcohol had many names, which caused some confusion; but by the 14th century, it would become known both as "wine" and "liquor" a migrating definition that would change to fit the purposes of governments.

In 1828, Noah Webster provided a dictionary definition calling liquor "the most common application is to spirituous fluids, whether distilled or fermented, to decoctions, solutions or tinctures." This broad definition unfortunately merged "liquor" and "wine" into the same definition and category because they were both liquids and were classed as spirituous fluids even though wine was not distilled.

However, the public would come to know liquor as alcoholic drinks which included liquor, wine and beer that were fermented but never distilled. Even a child knows these are not the same. This same definition remains in the 21st century dictionaries.

The "bomb blast" began worldwide confusion because distilled spirits at the family dinner table and for Communion created a drunken condition for the Christians. Drunkenness was quickly regarded by the Catholic Church as "natural" and a blameless condition.[33] Drunkenness, both at the dinner tables and at Communion in the churches, where "strong drink" was now a product of the past, dominated the Christian culture as Rome claimed to have the only church. Communion moved among the priests where liquor created drunkenness and chaos around their tables and created a scandalous heritage of immorality within the Church.

At a time in history in which wines were seven to ten percent alcohol with unstable shelf lives, a substance was distilled from wine (brandy) or beer (spirits) that caused it to have unlimited shelf life, get people drunk quickly, and it was just in time to replace the European vineyards that were freezing out from what has become known as the "Little Glaciation Period" also "Little Ice Age." Most important, grain fermentation would produce less costly liquor than grape fermentation. Distillation changed the world of chemistry. Lull had found 65% alcohol, and even technology that could take it to 97%, which immediately was mixed with wine to stop weak and feeble wines from going bad before Communion. It was cheap and profitable for the Church which became a world supplier.

A new culture was created so that when spirits were added to the mixing bowl the four-to-one mixture assured everyone who drank the new wine got drunk, from children and mothers, to saints in the Church. Lull's embellishment would start 800 years of a "Drunk Fad" a "Bomb Blast," and *destruction to the medical technologies* for using real wine. The books of medicine changed from those of Hippocrates to *The Great Book of Distillation* in 1552, which mainly replaced wine with liquor treatments.

No explanations were made by doctors for why liquor did not work, but drunken patients did not care so much and the new MDs accepted this as proof of proper treatment. It was a preferable treatment because the patients came back as drunks and remained alcoholic patients for life. The doctor's prescription made drunkenness a sanctified way of life. The words "cure" and "heal" as the result of medical treatment would become hotly debated until the twenty-first century when the word would not be used at all as a result of medical treatment. The argument was that the "body healed itself" and the doctors only provided "treatments". The doctor could not cure a person, the body cured itself. The dictionaries would redefine the words "heal" and "cure" as "treatment" which broke the pledge of the Hippocratic Oath that the doctor healed patients. The MDs required less medical education than the DOs of ancient history and the Great Book of Distillation became the MDs treatment system, a system accused of keeping the patients drunk and not healing them. Liquor would herein divide the medical world.

Iain Gately comprehensively reported in his book *DRINK, A Cultural History of Alcohol,* which gives the global impact of the discovery of liquor. Gately reports that "only the wealthy and the church could afford wine."[34] However, everyone could afford burnt water (liquor distilled from grains) and the new liquor was able to absorb many flavors that wine would overpower with its own flavor, which was desired for water purification and taking bitter herbs. During the 1800s each nation began producing its own national liquor drink and flavors. America went to whiskey and bourbon; England had gin; France took up cognac and brandy; then there was Caribbean rum, Japanese sake and rice wine, Chinese wine, Irish scotch, and Russian vodka all made into nationalistic drinks from fermented carbohydrates, which distinguished nations and multiplied the nationalistic drunkenness fads.

Wine had truly been swallowed into oblivion as the culture of drunkenness exploded. This fad burdened society to accept drunks as a part of the mainstream of culture. Fatal accidents and immoral abuse caused by the drunks was tolerated, as great leaders of the churches agreed drunkenness was favored by God. Laws could not undo what historians would call a "spiritual curse" upon mankind by the unknowing Catholic Church.

To gain understanding of the world views of liquor, Gately researched the attitudes of nations as the practice of intoxication became a world epidemic by the thirteenth century. It endured some 800 years from roughly 1300 until the present with the intermission of Prohibition in some nations, at which time religions began to teach against "all spirits." But, during this time it was fashionable for men, children, and women to be drunk. The Biblical laws against drunkenness were compromised. International church leadership claimed it was a good thing to get drunk and the church used liquor in Communion cups.

The liquor bomb produced addicts formerly called drunkards, perhaps in a great spiritual war upon the earth because liquor replaced strong drink. Nations of alcoholics resulted. Alcoholics Anonymous would start up acknowledging the significance that alcoholism could not be cured physically and it was a spiritual disease that required salvation. After years of questionable success, salvation was removed from the program by demand of other religions. They began calling God a "higher power" so drunks from all religions could participate. The historical documentation of AA has found that not one person has remained an active participant in the meeting program for life, as intended. The program is designed where no one is ever allowed to be freed from alcohol and must confess at every meeting, "I am an alcoholic" which is a spiritual curse. By claiming the curse repeatedly to be an alcoholic, the drunks are never allowed to recover or be free of alcoholism. Herein they soon learn AA will never let them be free and discontinue attendance.

The psychology industry started in 1950 at the universities to deal with alcoholism without salvation and entered into a drug world of addictions claiming alcoholism was just one of many. Food addiction, drug addiction, sex addiction, gambling addiction, sweets addiction, stock market addiction, golf addiction, and anything that dominated a person's activities became a recognized addiction worthy of hospitalization with insurance payments. Research claims the addictions are not the same, but they are compulsive behavior over which individuals fail to take control and psychology is struggling to provide an answer. Perhaps repetition of anything does create the habit, such as safety training of a pilot which creates automatic responses without thinking, or even driving a car. Auto behavior can be good or bad. Repetition of drinking the same beverage does create the habit from coco and coffee to coca cola or wine, or liquor, or beer. Those habits that are destructive to other people are crimes. Habits destructive to oneself can be deadly. So how does society retrain or break habits? This successful system has not been created. Laws definitely do not break habits.

Modern research continues to open new light upon wine; its nutrition, its medical properties, and the purposes of God to establish the foundation of world health upon the pillars of wine. Both God and Christ have established habits of drinking wine as a foundation of religion. Wine was the first food given to a starving man in early history. It was the traditional food when churches were hospitals. Hospitals in the West do not give wine to patients as a rebellion against alcohol. Nobody explained to the American people that distilled alcohol was thought to be a "super wine" in 1225 when it was discovered. The Biblical characteristics of strong drink were redefined by the Pope to be distilled spirits, liquor, or alcohol. Spirits did not have vitamins, minerals, enzymes or acids, as strong drink did, because it was distilled out of the foods. The more pure the alcohol, the more water that was separated from it but no minerals or acids would survive the first distillation. Spirits had none of the good stuff of nutrition.

Strong drink on the other hand was the king of nutrition and backbone of the Hebrew culture. In Patrick McGovern's book *Ancient Wine, the Search for the Origins of Viniculture*, he has documented the cultures of kingdoms, many tombs, pottery in museums, and tested the types of wines the kings used. Having tested the wines of thousands of pots with sophisticated electronic sampling technology his remarks about the wines of the Hebrew families were very interesting. "The wine is always 'old wine,' presumably well-aged vintage, and the olive oil is exclusively 'washed oil' likely a cold pressed, filtered fraction of the highest quality."[35] "Old wine" would be called "strong drink" in Hebrew culture. McGovern's mission is to discover the ancient grapes, the original viniculture of Noah, and as result he may be the most knowledgeable person worldwide about grape types and purity of wines.

Liquor destroyed wine cultures because it was brought into the Catholic Church "as a new blessing from God." Cultures were destroyed by drunks, who had the blessings of the Church. The Church created the drunks, many of whom were priests. Priests could drink strong drink and wine without getting drunk only by repetitious training and discipline, but the new "aqua vita" made them drunk quickly. Addiction became a church-approved condition internally and externally, while societies suffered. Drunkenness became a Church benefit as lands worldwide would be given up to the Church by drunks, in a culture that caused Martin Luther to be the first to break from the Church because of its ethical misbehavior. The Dark Ages always had drunks in literature because the Church approved of them, even believed they were proof of righteous living and being honest with God. Alcoholism was a playground.

When the American churches learned they had been deceived by liquor, they threw out the wine with the liquor in Prohibition. They threw out God's blessing. They threw out the "remember me" part of the New Testament quote of Christ. This research has provided the opportunity to learn important history about wine, and I am finding even the churches have no idea why or how they quit using wine for Communion. They have no concept it is important to use real wine with a real Christ. There is no such thing as a substitute wine. Make believe was not part of Christ's blood covenant in the New Testament. John Wesley was the first to defend wine from the damages of liquor. He separated definitions.

John Wesley "Freedom from Liquor and Addiction"

After 517 years, the world had discovered the curse of drunkenness was not a blessing as the Catholic and Anglican Churches pretended. John Wesley started the dynamic Methodist Churches by fighting against drunkenness and exposing the fraud. He led the churches and nations against the Catholic and Anglican Church laws that blessed being drunk. Drunkenness had become a culture in which the drunk had church protection and authority where even murder was not a capital crime. "Intent" is still the difference between murder and manslaughter in Western law. This was a great legal problem between the Colonies and Indian Tribes where the Indians innately applied the laws that they had to get drunk before avenging a wrong. However, the Colonies refused to apply this law to Indian murders. The law says a man must be of sound mind to commit murder, and drunkenness is legal proof that the man "could not have had intent."

Drunkenness gave good reason to homosexual acts, rapes, and wife or child abuses.

Entering the Dark Ages, liquor had the reputation of a saint. That reversed with John Wesley, as the people were no longer deceived that God blessed drunks or what would later be called addicts. There was no nutrition in gin or biblical reason to use it for Communion Wine. Wesley kept grape wine for Communion, which had nutrition. Wesley rejected and preached against the blessings of liquor by the Angleton High Priest and Pope. Wesley began his "fire and brimstone" ministry in 1742 and by 1750 he had reduced the gin consumption of England by 85%. The Angleton Church stood against this upstart, who was preaching against the "Drunk Fad," which was approved by the Anglican Bishop and Catholic Pope. Barred from the Anglican Churches, even though his father was a high Priest at Oxford University, and his two brothers where respected priests Wesley held "open air" and "home church" revivals where he preached to tens of thousands that gin was evil and destroyed lives. The public agreed with him. His sermons were brilliant and he taught abstinence from gin, which ranged upward to 65% distilled alcohol. However, he magnified the difference between gin and wine by insisting on drinking natural wine for Church Communion. He taught that the Churches had mixed the definitions of wine. According to Dr. Brewer, "natural wine defined in the Bible as strong wine or strong drink could not have produced more than thirteen percent alcohol and more typically was close to seven percent because the climate was cold. Even adding raisins or sugars could not raise the levels yeast would produce. Anything higher than 13% had to be distilled."

Beginning in 1742 John Wesley led what has to be called a spiritual battle against gin, which was being consumed at about one-fourth cup per day for every man, woman, and child in England. This created a drunken and highly immoral nation. Drunkenness and immorality are indeed spiritual partners. He started the Methodist Church in which every person had to be a teetotaler to join. Even better, and to the chagrin of the Catholic and Anglican Leadership, he appointed thousands of Methodist lay pastors who opened thousands of Methodist Churches worldwide and led a religious revolution that required all members to swear against distilled alcohol.[36] Wine did not include liquor in the same definition in Wesley's Church. [37]

I am confident that Wesley had no history about how the Catholic Church entangled liquor into the Communion Cup and blessed the drunks. The Catholic Church would become the "Father of Alcohol Addiction." Information was not available about the Alembic Still history and the Catholic Church records were not available for scholars. However, Wesley knew the Bible spoke against drunkenness and yet the Pope and High Priest shielded drunks. This was not Biblical.

Wesley was the first to stand against the Catholic and Anglican Churches using teetotalism as a weapon. Biblical wine was not restored in the Churches, but scientific instruments were not yet available to discover the difference in alcohol content. However, the pastors were confused worldwide over the definition of wine. Wesley was making a distinction between natural wine for Communion and liquor for drunkenness. Methodists removed the drunks and liquor from the churches. It may be more proper to give him credit for breaking the back of addiction as he dried out hundreds of thousands of drunks and restored their dignity. Perhaps his success is the only program that has wiped out alcoholism, and hundreds of programs have failed.

Wesley naturally brought his campaign to America where he was received with great blessings by many church leaders. America stood up in rebellion against drunkenness and liquor all in one movement. Wesley was a smashing success but was standing against Anglican churches in America, and did not receive his blessings with open arms. He may have brought the roots of prohibition to

America in the late 1700s. It was a rebellion in which any housewife who loved her family could support. Liquor had ruled the world long enough and the Churches were wrong to use liquor in Communion. It was not God's plan according to Methodists. The seeds of abolishing liquor were planted.

With the Catholic and Anglican Churches fatally flawed, the Methodists crawled across America with emphasis on reading their Bibles and becoming leaders. Hundreds of secular churches would rise up to join the spiritual warfare. Liquor banning was on the mind of a nation, but the real wine was the very thing liquor claimed to be by the Church definition. So, lack of a definition for wine by Christ and God that separated it from liquor would throw a nation into Prohibition. The notion arose that the church should choose between "Bad Wine," which makes a man drunk vs. "Good Wine," which does not. Reverend Edward H. Jewett saw an opportunity to clarify God's intention.

Wesley remained faithful to wine Communion and taught all his ministers to do the same, however, they would forget the foundational rule of teetotalism that established Methodists after he was gone. They would replace Communion wine with pasteurized grape juice.

The Debate of "Good Wine" vs. "Bad Wine" in 1882

The original story is that on December 28, 1882, Reverend Edward H. Jewett had 264 out of 286 clergymen assembled for the new Society of Biblical Literature vote to stop using all liquor or "Bad Wine" for Communion[38] and to use the pasteurized grape juice as a substitute that Pasteur had just invented as good wine. Regrettably twenty-two pastors could not stop the destruction of wine for Communion, as if God's will was determined by these votes of men. It seems that only the Catholics and a couple of small churches survived the test and continued using real wine for Communion. This Society was only twelve-years old, but it electrified the US Christian world with a debate that continues to unravel today and demanded a "substitute wine" for Communion with Christ. They still have not learned the Hebrews mixed strong drink one to four with water and had no place for a substitute wine as the wine mixture they drank was roughly two percent alcohol.

Can we believe Merriam Webster's definition that there can be "a substitute" for wine? Can there be a phony liquid, a make believe, a dead substance devoid of wine's nutrition used for Communion? I guess there can since the other modern dictionaries say the same thing. Liquor was the "first substitute" for strong drink back in 1225, approved by a Pope, but it was believed to be a "super wine substitute". For 800 years, the Catholic Church has used a "substitute" for wine in Communion, but they were deceived into believing it was truly wine. Nobody wants to reverse a Pope's Bulls. But here was an American organization leading the pastors from 100% liquor for wine to 100% make believe of wine using cooked juice.

In 1886, only four years after Jewett's meeting, the Catholics partly honored the Jewett decision with a new Bull. They cut back the alcohol content in Communion to a maximum of eighteen percent alcohol, which could save weak wine production from grapes that did not yield ten percent alcohol. The Catholic Church Bull agreed to cut back the alcohol content but still use liquor to beef up its wine, a commercial function for saving the Communion wine industry. The weak wines came from weak natural yeasts, but also processing the juice before grapes are ripe, which is a major problem for machine grape picking and cold climate grapes. Once the natural fermentation is altered, does it make any difference what the alcohol content is? The Church is going to change this Bull again a hundred years later in 1986. The impact of watching the Church change universal laws lets mankind see that nothing man does is reliable, and only God's laws do not change.

It is my suspicion that since we have been learning from Agnes Morgan since 1938 that fermented wine has a powerhouse of nutritional and medical benefits, surely Christ knew what he was doing when he told his disciples to "drink ye all of it" as Matthew reported. Was he making sure they gained a physical benefit and would pass his instructions to followers? If his Church drank a four ounce cup of wine daily, don't you think he knew he was giving them health? Telling them to "do this in remembrance of me" would not have much nutritional power if "a little sip would do". However, if it was drunk at every meal as a cultural habit, it would have great nutritional impact.

His instruction was for home-table Communion, as well as for Church leaders; however, it made a great difference when liquor rendered Communion a drunken event instead of just remembering Christ. Can you imagine the reaction of the first priest that had to serve liquor to hundreds at the rate of a four ounce cup each? So perhaps the economics of wine is the reason the cups turned to sips. However, it could be because they got drunk during Communion or just used too much wine. No question about it, if all the Christians drank four ounces of wine a day for health, the Christian world would be a powerhouse of healthy people. Can you imagine the power they would have in governments or whatever they set their collective minds to do?

The American churches created the second change in definition of "strong drink" out of the Jewett Debate on "Good Wine vs. Bad Wine". "Bad Wine" made one drunk and "Good Wine" did not. The Bible definitely warns about getting drunk on strong drink and as the Greeks told us, wine was its own judge, jury, and penalty for over-indulging offenders. These church fathers did not want liquor in their Communion cups and did not want drunkards in the families. Their intentions are clear.

Jewett's "Bad Wine" included the liquor definition of wine that ranged from zero to 65 percent alcohol. "Good Wine" could not have any alcohol in it at all and, therefore, could not make a man drunk. "Good Wine" did not include the definition of the Greeks or Hebrews of a one-part strong drink to four-parts water mixture. The records of Scripture quoted demonstrate Jewett did not know about the Hebrews mixing water to make wine at the 1.2% to 2.4% alcohol levels. American churches did not use wine to purify water; they had pure water from wells and springs. Purifying water with wine was never an American custom. The problem was how to throw off the yoke of the Pope and just return to Biblical wine.

The American culture in 1882 was a liquor-based culture of whiskey and white lightening, but the worldwide definition of wine allowed both to be called wine. Jewett's "Good Wine" definition only debated grape juice that could be boiled to stop the fermentation process before it turned into strong drink by the fermentation of sugar contained in every grape. The Bible never mentioned good or bad wine or canned juice. The whole debate was an attempt to separate wine from liquor, but they did not succeed. The research instruments were not available to show how much alcohol was in a drink or if it had vitamins and minerals. However, the Scriptures were dissected to discover the places where fresh juice was drunk in the Bible and those used for Jewett's decision—but wait there is a deception in the decision.

Louis Pasteur died in 1895 and had just published his research on pasteurization of wine to stop it from going bad. The USDA had just started requiring pasteurization of milk to destroy brucellosis. The decision must have seemed to the pastors to have been brought to them by God with the new pasteurization process just dropped in their laps. WOW! New technology regarding wine was totally misunderstood a second time. Only this time it is the reverse of the first error. They have moved from up to 97% levels of alcohol to zero percent, neither of which is wine established by both God and Christ at the one to one mixture of strong drink and water, which ranges from 3.5% alcohol to 6.5% at the maximum levels. However, the Hebrew mixture level was traditionally one to four which ranges down to 1.4% for 7% strong drink and 2.6% for 13%

strong drink.

So first we have drunken Christians trying to commune with the Lord on "liquor substitutes" make believe that has no meaning, no nutrition. Now we have the church turning away from wine totally and drinking juice substitutes. Liquor has no life. Pasteurized grape juice has no life. Wine has life.

The Society of Biblical Literature chose to use grape juice that was boiled to kill the natural yeast, which would then not ferment into wine used for Communion.[39] I have heard it argued many times that "the wine is only symbolic" so that makes it okay. One pastor in Jewett's meeting reported using water for Communion wine instead of liquor. One reported placing the wine and bread on a table so the members could walk by and observe the wine and bread as remembrance. As we saw in the Hebrew definitions, even the fresh squeezed juice has a special name in the Bible; however, there was not a "wine substitute" provided, as Merriam Webster called it. Jewett's pastors did not acknowledge that God provided the yeast in each grape by design to make it ferment into wine. Without fermentation hundreds of acids and vitamins would not be in the wine. There would not be a nutrition or medical benefit, as one found in the real wine. At least the Catholic Church did not claim a substitute for wine and they still drink real wine for Communion today. Still, we recognize the Catholic Church had again been deceived regarding Communion when they changed the Bull in 1886 to no more than eighteen percent alcohol wine. I am currently researching *Wine's Communion Power,* which will reveal more of Rev. Jewett's politics behind "Good Wine vs. Bad Wine."

The Essential Vine

With this research, we still have not considered the great value of the grapevine itself in giving us nutrition. Christ had a lot to say about the vine. Is there something critical about the grapevine that has been hidden from public knowledge? There is.

Wine has no contamination attached to it. It is a pure drink from the vine filtration system. The grapevine root filters out the contamination in the water from bacteria, fungus, nuclear fallout, diseases, and chemicals.

WOW! The root filtration of a grapevine system grows to depths from five to fifty feet—deep enough to reach the underground water table chocked full of minerals. Are you as astounded as I am at how the minerals come up into the grape clusters from underground water tables? It supplies nutrition while filtering out diseases to the juices. This is masterful if not miraculous. Many of the modern agriculture vineyards are backed up with public watering systems acclaimed to be the state of the art in agriculture. These systems result in shallow roots for the vines that are dependent upon man's management, but they do control production. These watering methods can deliver fertilizer and chemical fungicides systemically, which is scientific. So as we look back to history for our guidelines, man did not have chlorine-based public watering systems or runoff ponds of pesticides to yield contamination to the vines. These are not the vines of history that went fifty feet to a water table. However, even when vines are assaulted with diseases and chemicals, the roots still purify the juice.

Wine is the primary choice for a safe drink worldwide which explains the Biblical social customs of offering wine to refresh a guest. The vineyards qualify to be God's greatest blessing to man's health by bringing a pure and nutritious drink for thirst. The vine is an integral part of the power of wine as it delivers unadulterated blessings. It would be devastating to go through disaster and have no wine to purify the water of cholera, typhus and brucellosis as happened to the British Army when Nightingale saved them.

Fine Dining

There really is such a thing as fine dining and many people have it in their homes. It does include decorum in fine taste, table clothes, wine and thousands of chef's specials. Chinese took me to a special dinner every night and called it a banquet. As a General Manager or President of a manufacturing company I had sort of a War Lord status the Chinese understand and honor with fine dining and everyone said "yes" in public conversation. America does not have family traditions, or better as in China, government traditions for dining. That was my first experience to discover that wine at a banquet was always what Americans call straight liquor of a 40-55% alcohol. It was always made from grain. They did have grape wine but it had no status for executive dining and I never saw it on the table of the highest officers which ranged from mayors, to province leaders, to county judges or industrial leaders.

After learning about wine many people want to add wine to their diet and ask me "What is the best wine to drink?" I tell them that they are almost equally good because they are a "fermented nutrient rich drink." The nutrition and medical benefits come from the fermentation process. It makes no difference if it is the most expensive or least expensive, the oldest or the newest, the sweetest or the driest, they will have a similar nutrition benefit. I do drink a sweet wine with sugars to recover when I am exhausted. However, I normally drink a red wine. I have drunk many wines I did not like very well and would not put into my collection. However, some of my friends loved the ones I did not prefer. You will discover that people have a wide variation of tastes they like. The Chinese had a salt based food system and loved dried fish while Americans generally have a sugar based system that favored sweet dishes. Many tastes are commonly liked, and many are commonly disliked. This is not a universal science, but most wine is sold for flavor.

Resveratrol in the wines are elevating the values of wine today. The resveratrol is highest in red wines, perhaps as much as eight times the white wines as reported. However, this spread is not the same as typical vitamins, minerals, enzymes, or acids which seldom vary over 20%. Out of 3,400 research studies performed, all of which found major benefits in the wine, none gave a test of the perhaps hundreds of types of grapes available to analyze. The prices of wine typically are based upon supply and demand by different wineries and some raise prices by advertising and reputation, but you should find a wine or wines you like and stick to them. Good wineries have oversupply problems occasionally and must put their inventory on "special" in order to bring in ripe fields. If you know their wines, you will be able to stock up when this happens.

I like the Muscadine wine best and elderberry/blackberry fits my taste. I like wines that are unmixed because so many mixed wines have sulfites that were added to stop the oxidation when the bottle is corked. Invariably, I think I can taste the sulfite; but my friend, Dr. John Brewer, who is a judge for wine competitions, tells me the only reason that happens is because the wine master did not know what he was doing when he added too much sulfite. Dr. Brewer claims he can tell whether the problem is the wine master, the corks, or the grapes. He reported there should be a 30-to-40-parts-per-million sulfite in the bottle and you should never taste it. I have no doubt there are many untrained wine masters out there.

My water filtration engineer tells me my water has about one-part-per-million and never over four-parts-per-million chlorine, and sometimes I can taste and smell it. John says the headaches or allergies of wine typically come from a mold, but people are not allergic to the wine. They are allergic to something that should not be there. He says you should follow the Wine Master in selecting wines. I can testify there is something for decision making in all that he says. It changes my whole attitude toward choosing wine. I am trying to start my own Muscadine arbor and like my friend who gets 250 gallons from a patch about 20 x 40 feet I will be very pleased if that little patch produces what I like. However, Glenda Sue likes too many varieties of wine to plan for her so I need some friends who will trade.

I believe wine is God's Biblical provision. I drink four to five ounces (maybe more) each day and start an hour to twenty minutes before dinner. The 1,000 acids and many enzymes in wine become my major digestion system, instead of causing my body to produce hydrochloric acid. This produces a more complete digestion and purifies all foods of bacteria. It encourages joyful dining and sociability. I like peace and the wine is a moment of sharing with Glenda Sue. The bottom line is that it is the people that make fine dining and I think the dining establishes a family peace. Perhaps strangely, it causes us to remember the words that were spoken 2,000 years ago. Every time we share the wine, we invariably toast "To the Lord!" I believe this was Christ's intention. Stay healthy! Drink wine for your health, enjoyment, and to "Remember Him!"

ENDNOTES

1 Oribasius, Athenaeus. Quotes Mnesitheus of Athens: *Medical Collection*.4th Century BC. (http://www.mlahanas.de /Greeks/ Bios /MnesitheusOfAthens.html).

2 Magiera, Janet M. Aramaic Peshitta New Testament Parallel Translations. (KJV, Murdock, Magiera). Deuteronomy 7:13. July 13, 2005.

3 Ibid.

4 Brewer, John PhD, Owner. Wyldwood Cellars Winery. Personal Interview. May 25, 2014.

5 Morgan, Agnes Fay, Tielen I. Nobles, Adina Wiens, George L. Marsh and Albcst J. Winkles. The B Vitamins of California Grape Juices and Wine. Laboratories of Home Economics, Fruit Products, and Viticulture. College of Agriculture. University of California, Berkley and Davis, CA. Food Research Volume 4, No.3. Revised for Publication. October 24, 1938.

6 Wikipedia. Acids in Wine. (Internet, 2010).

7 Wikipedia. French Wine Guide. Wine Component/Composition of Wine. (Internet, 2010).

8 SR-21. Nutritional Information on Alcoholic Beverage. U.S. Government Regulations. Wine Table Red. *USDA* 1976.

9 Brewer, John PhD. July 8, 2011.

10 Pezzuto, John M., PhD. UIC. Plant-Derived Anticancer Agents. *Biochem. Pharmacol.* 53: 121–133, 1997.

11 Jang, M., Cai, L., Udeani, G.O., slowing, K., Thomas, C.F., Beecher, C.W.W., Fong, H.H.S., Farnsworth, N.R., Kinghorn, A.D., Mehta, R.G., Moon, R.C., and Pezzuto, J.M. Cancer chemopreventive activity of resveratrol, a natural product derived from grapes. *Science*. 275: 218–220. 1997.

12 Penumathsa, S. V. and Maulik, N. Resveratrol: A Promising Agent in Promoting Cardio Protection against Coronary Heart Disease. *US National Library of Medicine*, April 2009.

13 Vogalman, Ryan. How Resveratrol Combats Leading Causes of Death. *Life Extension Magazine*. March 2012.

14 Guerra, Bilblana. Wine Antioxidants: Understanding the Basics of Phenolic Compounds. *Wine Business Monthly*. July 15, 2008.

15 Agriculture Marketing Service. National Organic Program. *USDA*. 2012.

16 McGovern, Patrick E.. Ancient Wine: the Search for the Origins of Viniculture. (Princeton: University Press. 2003).

17 Campbell, Colin T. PhD. & Thomas M. Campbell II, MD. The China Study: The most comprehensive study of nutrition ever conducted. (Dallas: Benbella Books. 2006).

18 Oribasius. "Athenaeus quotes Mnesitheus of Athens." *Medical Collection*. 4th Century BC. http://www.mlahanas.de /Greeks/ Bios/MnesitheusOfAthens.html

19 American Dictionary of the English Language. Noah Webster. Facsimile First Edition. (San Francisco: Foundation for American Christian Education. 1928).

20 Merriam Webster's Collegiate Dictionary, Tenth Edition. (Springfield Merriam-Webster, Inc.1994).

21 Brewer, John, PhD. March 3, 2010.

22 Leary, T. The Therapeutic Value of Wine. *BioOne Online Journals PubMed, CSA*. Liquor & Cardio-Vascular Health: Wine, Liquor, Beer, and Mortality. *American Journal of Epidemiology*. 158:585–95, 1931.

23 Norrie, P.A., Wine: A Scientific Exploration, The History of

Wine as a Medicine II, 1941. 50.

24 Jacob Gaffney. Scientists Move to Harness Red Wine Compound's Power. *Advances in Experimental Medicine and Biology.* 2008.

25 Images of Food Pyramids of the World. World Wide Web. *Google* 2013.

26 Norrie, P.A.. Wine: A Scientific Exploration. The History of Wine as a Medicine II. 1941. 28.

27 Kappagoda, C. T. Cardiologist. University of California, Davis. Research Paper: Red Wine Dilates Blood Vessels. Experimental Biology 98. *American Psychological Society.* 1998.

28 Beeson, W. Dr. University of Kentucky. Unidentified Growth Factors in Distiller's Grains. Research Report: National Distiller's Convention. Louisville, KY. 1970.

29 Norrie, P.A. Wine: A Scientific Exploration. The History of Wine as a Medicine II. 1941. 50.

30 Wikipedia. French Wine Guide: Wine Component/Composition of Wine. 2010.

31 Renaud, Serge, Dr. French Paradox. 60 Minutes. 1991.

32 Gately, Iain. DRINK. A Cultural History of Alcohol. Gotham Books. 2008. 72.

33 Gately, Iain. DRINK. 76.

34 Ibid.

35 McGovern, Patrick E. Ancient Wine: The Search for the Origins of Viniculture (Princeton: University Press). 2007.

36 Meredith, William. The Real John Wesley, Jennings & Pye. 1903. 227.

37 Brewer, John, PhD. March 3, 2010.

38 Jewett, Edward H, Rev., DD, LLD. The Two Wine Theory. Communion Wine. 5th Edition. (Park Place: New York & Co 25. 1890.

39 Ibid.

Review Requested:
If you loved this book, would you please provide a review at Amazon.com?